Menu
type 2 diabetes cookbook for 1 person

Breakfast Recipes for Blood Sugar Control

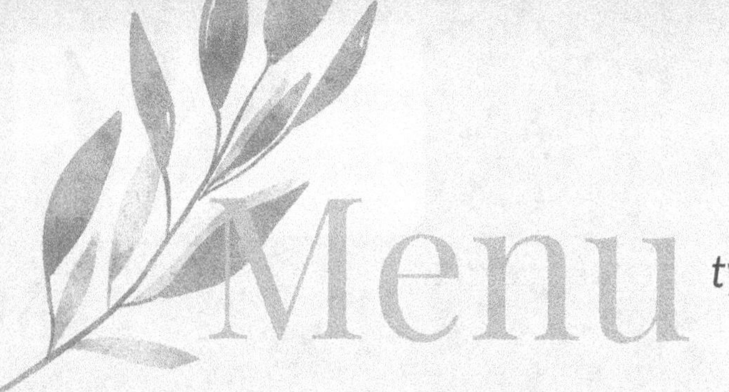

Menu

*type 2 diabetes cookbook for
1 person*

Lunch Recipes for Sustained Energy

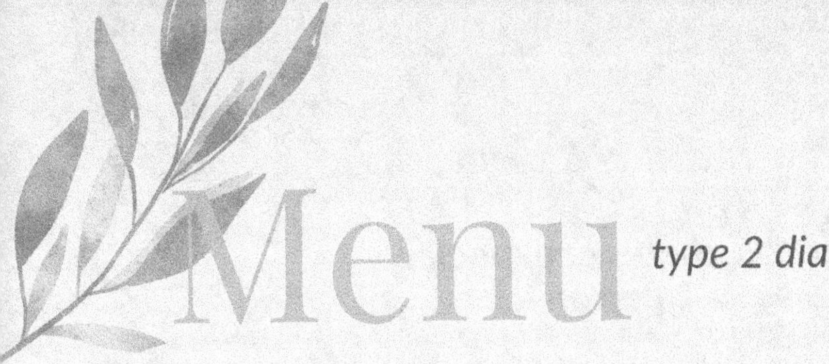

Menu

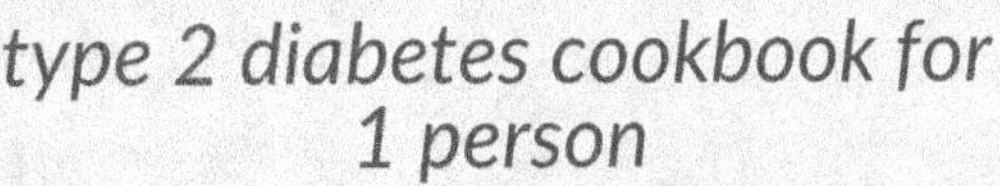

*type 2 diabetes cookbook for
1 person*

Dinner Recipes for Balanced Nutrition

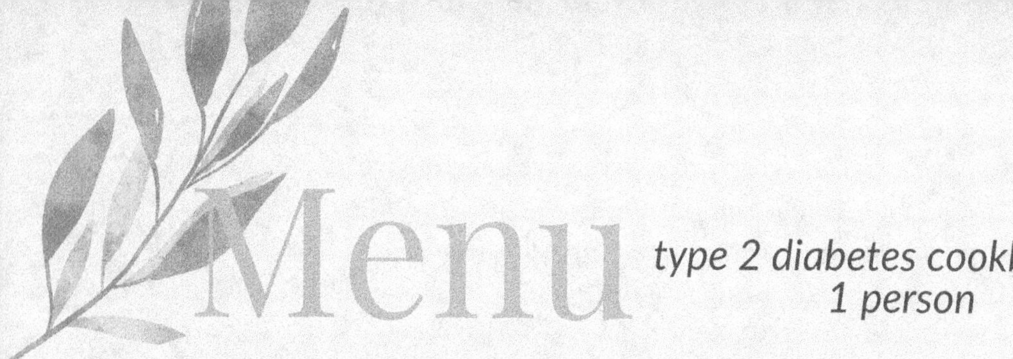

Menu

type 2 diabetes cookbook for 1 person

Snack Ideas to Keep Blood Sugar Stable

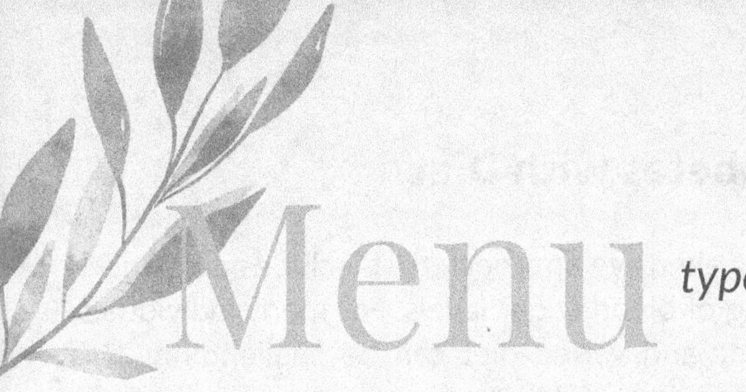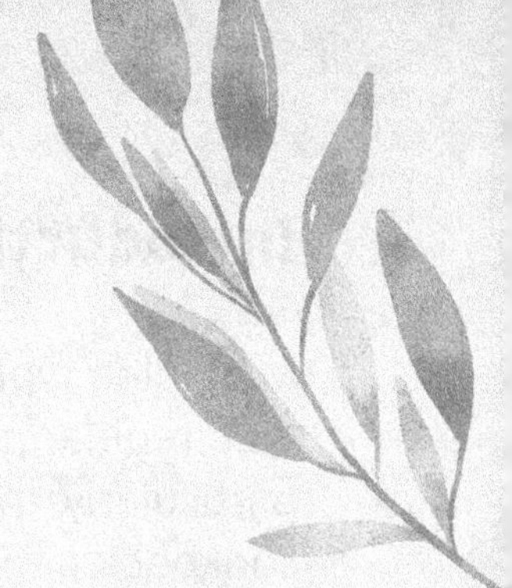

Menu
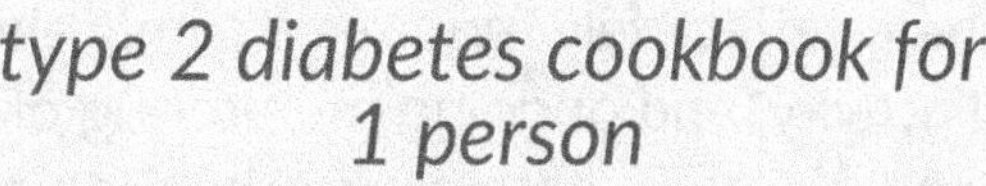
type 2 diabetes cookbook for 1 person

Desserts that Won't Spike Your Blood Sugar

Introduction to Managing Type 2 Diabetes with Diet

Managing type 2 diabetes effectively requires a comprehensive approach that includes a balanced diet, regular physical activity, and ongoing monitoring of blood sugar levels. For many individuals, particularly those living alone, maintaining a healthy and varied diet can be challenging. This cookbook aims to simplify the process by providing a variety of delicious, easy-to-prepare recipes tailored specifically for one person.

Understanding Type 2 Diabetes

Type 2 diabetes is a chronic condition characterized by insulin resistance, where the body's cells do not respond properly to insulin, leading to elevated blood sugar levels. Over time, high blood sugar can cause serious health complications, including heart disease, kidney damage, and nerve problems. However, with proper management, individuals with type 2 diabetes can lead healthy, fulfilling lives.

The Role of Diet in Diabetes Management

Diet plays a crucial role in managing type 2 diabetes. Eating the right foods can help control blood sugar levels, maintain a healthy weight, and prevent complications. Key dietary strategies include:

- Choosing Low Glycemic Index Foods: These foods cause a slower, more gradual rise in blood sugar levels.

- Balancing Macronutrients: Including a good mix of carbohydrates, proteins, and fats in every meal.

- Portion Control: Eating appropriate portion sizes to avoid overeating.

- Regular Meal Times: Eating at consistent times each day to help regulate blood sugar levels.

Challenges of Cooking for One

Cooking for one person presents unique challenges, such as food waste, difficulty in managing portion sizes, and lack of motivation to prepare meals. This cookbook addresses these issues by offering recipes that are specifically designed for single servings, reducing waste and making meal preparation more enjoyable.

How to Use This Cookbook

This cookbook is organized to provide comprehensive guidance on managing type 2 diabetes through diet. It starts with foundational knowledge on nutrition and essential kitchen tools, followed by chapters filled with recipes for breakfast, lunch, dinner, snacks, and desserts. Each recipe is crafted to be simple, nutritious, and suitable for one person. Additionally, chapters on meal planning, grocery shopping, and dining out provide practical tips to make healthy eating a seamless part of your daily routine.

Chapter 1: Understanding Nutritional Needs for Type 2 Diabetes

Effective management of type 2 diabetes begins with understanding your nutritional needs. This chapter delves into the specifics of how different nutrients affect blood sugar levels and overall health.

Macronutrients and Their Impact

- Carbohydrates: Carbohydrates have the most significant impact on blood sugar levels. Complex carbohydrates, such as whole grains and vegetables, are preferred because they digest more slowly, causing a gradual increase in blood sugar.

- Proteins: Protein helps stabilize blood sugar levels and keeps you feeling full. Including a source of protein in every meal is essential.

- Fats: Healthy fats, such as those found in nuts, seeds, and olive oil, are important for overall health and can help manage blood sugar levels.

Micronutrients and Their Importance

- Fiber: Fiber is crucial for managing blood sugar levels. It slows the absorption of sugar and can improve blood sugar control.

- Vitamins and Minerals: Certain vitamins and minerals, such as magnesium, chromium, and vitamin D, play roles in insulin sensitivity and glucose metabolism.

Creating a Balanced Plate

The concept of a balanced plate is a simple way to visualize a healthy meal. A balanced plate typically includes:

- Half non-starchy vegetables
- One-quarter lean protein
- One-quarter whole grains or starchy vegetables
- A small amount of healthy fat

Hydration and Blood Sugar Control

Staying hydrated is also important for managing blood sugar levels. Water is the best choice, but other beverages like herbal teas and unsweetened coffee can also be included.

Chapter 2: Essential Kitchen Tools and Ingredients

Having the right kitchen tools and ingredients can make preparing diabetes-friendly meals much easier. This chapter covers the essentials you need to stock your kitchen for success.

Must-Have Kitchen Tools
- Measuring Cups and Spoons: For accurate portion control.

- Food Scale: Helps with measuring portions, especially for items like meat and cheese.

- Blender or Food Processor: Useful for making smoothies, purees, and chopping vegetables.

- Non-Stick Skillet: Makes cooking with less oil possible.

- Sharp Knives and Cutting Board: Essential for efficient meal preparation.

Stocking Your Pantry
- Whole Grains: Brown rice, quinoa, whole wheat pasta.

- Legumes: Lentils, chickpeas, black beans.

- Nuts and Seeds: Almonds, chia seeds, flaxseeds.

- Healthy Oils: Olive oil, avocado oil.

- Low-Sodium Broth: For soups and stews.

- Herbs and Spices: To add flavor without extra calories or sodium.

Fresh Ingredients
- Non-Starchy Vegetables: Broccoli, spinach, bell peppers.

- Lean Proteins: Chicken breast, turkey, tofu.

- Fruits: Berries, apples, oranges (in moderation).

- Dairy or Dairy Alternatives: Low-fat yogurt, almond milk.

1. Spinach and Feta Omelette

Ingredients:
- 6 eggs
- 2 cups fresh spinach, chopped
- 1/2 cup crumbled feta cheese
- 2 tablespoons milk
- 1 tablespoon butter
- Salt and pepper to taste

PreparationTime: 10 minutes
Cook Time: 15 minutes
Total Time: 25 minutes
Serves: 2

Directions:

1. In a medium bowl, whisk the eggs, milk, salt, and pepper together until well combined.

2. Melt the butter in a non-stick skillet over medium heat.

3. Pour the egg mixture into the skillet and let it cook for 2-3 minutes, or until the edges start to set.

4. Sprinkle the chopped spinach and crumbled feta cheese over the top of the omelette.

5. Fold the omelette in half and continue cooking for another 2-3 minutes, or until the omelette is cooked through.

6. Slide the omelette onto a plate and serve hot.

Storage Instructions:

- Leftovers can be stored in an airtight container in the refrigerator for up to 3 days.

Variations and Tips:

- You can use other types of cheese, such as cheddar or goat cheese, instead of feta.
- Add diced tomatoes, mushrooms, or onions to the omelette for extra flavor.
- Serve the omelette with a side of toast or a small salad for a complete meal.

Nutrition Facts:

Calories: 280 | Total Fat: 19g | Saturated Fat: 9g | Cholesterol: 435mg | Sodium: 590mg | Total Carbohydrates: 6g | Dietary Fiber: 2g | Sugars: 2g | Protein: 22g

Breakfast Recipes for Blood Sugar Control

2. Greek Yogurt with Berries and Chia Seeds

Ingredients:
- 1 cup plain Greek yogurt
- 1/2 cup mixed berries
 (such as blueberries, raspberries, and blackberries)
- 1 tablespoon chia seeds

PreparationTime: 5 minutes
Cook Time: 0 minutes
Total Time: 5 minutes
Serves: 1

Directions:

1. In a bowl, combine the Greek yogurt, mixed berries, and chia seeds.

2. Stir gently to combine.

3. Serve immediately.

Storage Instructions:

- This dish can be stored in an airtight container in the refrigerator for up to 3 days.

Variations and Tips:

- You can use any type of berries you prefer, such as strawberries, blackberries, or a combination.

- Add a drizzle of honey or a sprinkle of cinnamon for extra flavor.

- For a crunchier texture, you can add chopped nuts or granola.

Nutrition Facts:

Calories: 220 | Total Fat: 8g | Saturated Fat: 3g | Cholesterol: 20mg | Sodium: 80mg | Total Carbohydrates: 18g | Dietary Fiber: 7g | Sugars: 11g | Protein: 20g

This recipe is a great option for managing type 2 diabetes because it is high in protein, fiber, and healthy fats, which can help regulate blood sugar levels and keep you feeling full and satisfied. The Greek yogurt provides a good source of protein, while the berries and chia seeds are rich in fiber and antioxidants. This dish can be enjoyed as a healthy snack or a light breakfast.

3. Oatmeal with Almond Butter and Sliced Bananas

Ingredients:
- 1/2 cup rolled oats
- 1 cup unsweetened almond milk
- 1 tablespoon almond butter
- 1 small banana, sliced
- 1 teaspoon cinnamon (optional)

PreparationTime: 5 minutes
Cook Time: 10 minutes
Total Time: 15 minutes
Serves: 1

Directions:

1. In a small saucepan, combine the rolled oats and almond milk.

2. Bring the mixture to a boil over medium heat, then reduce the heat and simmer for 5-7 minutes, stirring occasionally, until the oats are cooked and the mixture has thickened.

3. Remove the oatmeal from the heat and stir in the almond butter until well combined.

4. Top the oatmeal with the sliced banana and a sprinkle of cinnamon (if using).

Storage Instructions:

- Leftovers can be stored in an airtight container in the refrigerator for up to 3 days.

Variations and Tips:

- You can use any type of milk, such as cow's milk or soy milk, instead of almond milk.

- Add a handful of chopped nuts or a drizzle of honey for extra flavor and texture.

- For a creamier texture, you can mash the banana into the oatmeal before serving.

Nutrition Facts:

Calories: 330 | Total Fat: 14g | Saturated Fat: 1g | Cholesterol: 0mg | Sodium: 90mg | Total Carbohydrates: 45g | Dietary Fiber: 7g | Sugars: 12g | Protein: 10g

This recipe is a great option for managing type 2 diabetes because it is high in fiber, protein, and healthy fats, which can help regulate blood sugar levels and keep you feeling full and satisfied. The oats provide a slow-release of carbohydrates, while the almond butter and banana provide healthy fats and natural sweetness. This dish can be enjoyed as a nutritious breakfast or a filling snack.

4. Avocado Toast with Poached Egg

Ingredients:
- 2 slices whole-grain bread
- 1 ripe avocado, mashed
- 1 poached egg
- 1 tablespoon lemon juice
- Salt and pepper to taste

PreparationTime: 10 minutes
Cook Time: 5 minutes
Total Time: 15 minutes
Serves: 1

Directions:

1. Toast the whole-grain bread until lightly golden.

2. In a small bowl, mash the avocado with the lemon juice, salt, and pepper.

3. Spread the mashed avocado evenly over the toasted bread.

4. Carefully place the poached egg on top of the avocado toast.

Storage Instructions:

- This dish is best enjoyed immediately, as the poached egg and avocado will not keep well.

Variations and Tips:

- You can use different types of bread, such as sourdough or whole-wheat, for the toast.

- Add a sprinkle of red pepper flakes or a drizzle of olive oil for extra flavor.

- For a heartier meal, you can add sliced tomatoes, sautéed spinach, or crumbled feta cheese.

Nutrition Facts:

Calories: 320 | Total Fat: 18g | Saturated Fat: 3g | Cholesterol: 186mg | Sodium: 420mg | Total Carbohydrates: 28g | Dietary Fiber: 9g | Sugars: 3g | Protein: 13g

This recipe is a great option for managing type 2 diabetes because it is high in healthy fats, fiber, and protein, which can help regulate blood sugar levels and keep you feeling full and satisfied. The avocado provides healthy monounsaturated fats, while the whole-grain bread and poached egg provide a good source of complex carbohydrates and protein. This dish can be enjoyed as a nutritious breakfast or a light lunch.

5. Smoothie Bowl with Spinach, Avocado, and Flax Seeds

Ingredients:
- 1 cup unsweetened almond milk
- 1 cup fresh spinach
- 1/2 ripe avocado
- 1 frozen banana
- 1 tablespoon ground flax seeds
- 1 teaspoon honey (optional)

PreparationTime: 10 minutes
Cook Time: 0 minutes
Total Time: 10 minutes
Serves: 1

Directions:

1. In a high-speed blender, combine the almond milk, spinach, avocado, frozen banana, and flax seeds.

2. Blend the ingredients until smooth and creamy.

3. Pour the smoothie into a bowl and top with any desired toppings, such as additional fresh fruit, nuts, or a drizzle of honey (if using).

Storage Instructions:

- This smoothie bowl is best enjoyed immediately, as the avocado and spinach may not keep well if stored.

Variations and Tips:

- You can use any type of milk, such as cow's milk or soy milk, instead of almond milk.

- Add a scoop of protein powder or a tablespoon of nut butter for extra protein.

- Use a combination of frozen fruits, such as berries or mango, instead of just a banana.

- Top the smoothie bowl with crunchy toppings like granola, toasted coconut, or chopped nuts.

Nutrition Facts:

Calories: 350 | Total Fat: 18g | Saturated Fat: 2g | Cholesterol: 0mg | Sodium: 120mg | Total Carbohydrates: 40g | Dietary Fiber: 10g | Sugars: 16g | Protein: 8g

This smoothie bowl is an excellent option for managing type 2 diabetes because it is high in fiber, healthy fats, and antioxidants, which can help regulate blood sugar levels and support overall health. The spinach and avocado provide a nutrient-dense base, while the flax seeds and banana add natural sweetness and creaminess. This dish can be enjoyed as a nutritious breakfast or a satisfying snack.

Breakfast Recipes for Blood Sugar Control

6. Cottage Cheese with Fresh Peaches and Cinnamon

Ingredients:
- 1 cup low-fat cottage cheese
- 1 medium fresh peach, sliced
- 1/2 teaspoon ground cinnamon

PreparationTime: 5 minutes
Cook Time: 0 minutes
Total Time: 5 minutes
Serves: 1

Directions:

1. In a bowl, combine the cottage cheese and sliced peaches.

2. Sprinkle the ground cinnamon over the top.

3. Serve immediately.

Storage Instructions:

- This dish can be stored in an airtight container in the refrigerator for up to 3 days.

Variations and Tips:

- You can use any type of fresh fruit, such as berries, nectarines, or apricots, instead of peaches.

- Add a drizzle of honey or a sprinkle of chopped nuts for extra flavor and texture.

- For a creamier texture, you can blend the cottage cheese and peaches together before serving.

Nutrition Facts:

Calories: 200 | Total Fat: 4g | Saturated Fat: 2g | Cholesterol: 20mg | Sodium: 360mg | Total Carbohydrates: 18g | Dietary Fiber: 2g | Sugars: 14g | Protein: 22g

This recipe is a great option for managing type 2 diabetes because it is high in protein, low in added sugars, and provides a good source of fiber and antioxidants. The cottage cheese provides a good source of protein, while the fresh peaches and cinnamon add natural sweetness and flavor. This dish can be enjoyed as a healthy snack or a light breakfast.

7. Whole Grain Pancakes with Blueberries

Ingredients:
- 1 cup whole wheat flour
- 1 teaspoon baking powder
- 1/4 teaspoon baking soda
- 1/4 teaspoon salt
- 1 egg
- 1 cup unsweetened almond milk
- 1 tablespoon honey
- 1 cup fresh or frozen blueberries

PreparationTime: 10 minutes
Cook Time: 15 minutes
Total Time: 25 minutes
Serves: 2

Directions:

1. In a medium bowl, whisk together the whole wheat flour, baking powder, baking soda, and salt.

2. In a separate bowl, whisk the egg, almond milk, and honey until well combined.

3. Pour the wet ingredients into the dry ingredients and stir just until combined (do not overmix).

4. Fold in the blueberries.

5. Heat a non-stick skillet or griddle over medium heat. Scoop about 1/4 cup of the batter onto the hot surface and cook for 2-3 minutes, or until bubbles start to form on the surface.

6. Flip the pancake and cook for another 2-3 minutes, or until golden brown.

7. Repeat with the remaining batter, making about 8 pancakes total.

8. Serve the pancakes warm, with additional blueberries or a drizzle of honey if desired.

Storage Instructions:
- Leftover pancakes can be stored in an airtight container in the refrigerator for up to 3 days, or frozen for up to 3 months.

Variations and Tips:
- You can use other types of berries, such as raspberries or blackberries, instead of blueberries.
- Add a sprinkle of cinnamon or a tablespoon of chopped nuts for extra flavor and texture.
- Serve the pancakes with a side of Greek yogurt or a small salad for a more balanced meal.

Nutrition Facts:
Calories: 260 | Total Fat: 4g | Saturated Fat: 1g | Cholesterol: 55mg | Sodium: 390mg | Total Carbohydrates: 46g | Dietary Fiber: 5g | Sugars: 12g | Protein: 9g

This recipe is a great option for managing type 2 diabetes because it is made with whole grains, which provide a slow release of carbohydrates, and it is topped with fresh, fiber-rich blueberries. The addition of honey provides a natural sweetener, while the almond milk and egg add protein and healthy fats to help regulate blood sugar levels. These pancakes can be enjoyed as a nutritious breakfast or a satisfying snack.

Breakfast Recipes for Blood Sugar Control

8. Egg Muffins with Bell Peppers and Mushrooms

Ingredients:
- 8 large eggs
- 1/2 cup diced bell peppers (any color)
- 1/2 cup sliced mushrooms
- 2 tablespoons unsweetened almond milk
- 1/4 teaspoon salt
- 1/4 teaspoon black pepper

PreparationTime: 15 minutes
Cook Time: 25 minutes
Total Time: 40 minutes
Serves: 6 (1 muffin per serving)

Directions:

1. Preheat your oven to 350°F (175°C). Grease a 6-cup muffin tin with non-stick cooking spray or olive oil.

2. In a medium bowl, whisk the eggs, almond milk, salt, and black pepper until well combined.
3. Stir in the diced bell peppers and sliced mushrooms.

4. Divide the egg mixture evenly among the prepared muffin cups.

5. Bake for 20-25 minutes, or until the egg muffins are set and lightly golden on top.

6. Remove the muffin tin from the oven and let the egg muffins cool for 5 minutes before removing them from the tin. Serve the egg muffins warm.

Storage Instructions:
- Leftover egg muffins can be stored in an airtight container in the refrigerator for up to 4 days.

Variations and Tips:
- You can use any combination of vegetables, such as spinach, onions, or tomatoes, instead of or in addition to the bell peppers and mushrooms.
- Add a sprinkle of shredded cheese or a dollop of salsa on top of the egg muffins for extra flavor.
- Reheat the leftover egg muffins in the microwave or oven before serving.

Nutrition Facts:
Calories: 90 | Total Fat: 6g | Saturated Fat: 1g | Cholesterol: 185mg | Sodium: 210mg | Total Carbohydrates: 3g | Dietary Fiber: 1g | Sugars: 2g | Protein: 7g

These egg muffins are an excellent option for managing type 2 diabetes because they are high in protein, low in carbohydrates, and packed with nutrient-dense vegetables. The bell peppers and mushrooms provide fiber, vitamins, and antioxidants, while the eggs and almond milk offer a good source of healthy fats and protein to help regulate blood sugar levels. These muffins can be enjoyed as a quick and easy breakfast or a satisfying snack.

9. Chia Seed Pudding with Mixed Berries

Ingredients:
- 1/4 cup chia seeds
- 1 cup unsweetened almond milk
- 1 tablespoon honey (optional)
- 1/2 cup mixed berries (such as blueberries, raspberries, and blackberries)

PreparationTime: 10 minutes

Chilling Time: 2-4 hours

Total Time: 2-4 hours 10 minutes

Serves: 2

Directions:

1. In a medium bowl, whisk together the chia seeds and almond milk until well combined.

2. If using honey, stir it in now.

3. Cover the bowl and refrigerate for 2-4 hours, or until the chia seeds have thickened the mixture into a pudding-like consistency.

4. Divide the chia seed pudding into two serving bowls or jars.

5. Top each serving with 1/4 cup of the mixed berries.

Storage Instructions:

- The chia seed pudding can be stored in an airtight container in the refrigerator for up to 5 days.

Variations and Tips:

- You can use any type of milk, such as cow's milk or coconut milk, instead of almond milk.
- Add a sprinkle of cinnamon, a drizzle of vanilla extract, or a handful of chopped nuts for extra flavor and texture.
- For a creamier pudding, blend the chia seed mixture in a blender before chilling.

Nutrition Facts:

Calories: 180 | Total Fat: 9g | Saturated Fat: 1g | Cholesterol: 0mg | Sodium: 55mg | Total Carbohydrates: 20g | Dietary Fiber: 9g | Sugars: 10g | Protein: 5g

This chia seed pudding is an excellent option for managing type 2 diabetes because it is high in fiber, low in added sugars, and provides a good source of healthy fats and antioxidants. The chia seeds are a rich source of soluble fiber, which can help slow the absorption of carbohydrates and regulate blood sugar levels. The mixed berries add natural sweetness and a boost of vitamins and minerals. This dish can be enjoyed as a nutritious breakfast, snack, or dessert.

Breakfast Recipes for Blood Sugar Control

10. Quinoa Breakfast Bowl with Nuts and Seeds

Ingredients:
- 1/2 cup cooked quinoa
- 1/4 cup unsweetened almond milk
- 1 tablespoon chopped walnuts
- 1 tablespoon pumpkin seeds
- 1 tablespoon chia seeds
- 1 teaspoon honey (optional)
- 1/4 teaspoon ground cinnamon

PreparationTime: 10 minutes
Cook Time: 15 minutes
Total Time: 25 minutes
Serves: 1

Directions:

1. In a small saucepan, combine the cooked quinoa and almond milk. Heat over medium heat, stirring occasionally, until the mixture is warm and creamy, about 5 minutes.

2. Transfer the quinoa mixture to a bowl.

3. Top the quinoa with the chopped walnuts, pumpkin seeds, and chia seeds.

4. If desired, drizzle the honey over the top and sprinkle with the ground cinnamon.

Storage Instructions:

- Leftover quinoa can be stored in an airtight container in the refrigerator for up to 4 days.

Variations and Tips:

- Use any combination of nuts and seeds, such as almonds, pecans, or sunflower seeds.

- Add a spoonful of plain Greek yogurt or a sliced banana for extra protein and flavor.

- For a sweeter version, use vanilla-flavored almond milk or add a touch of maple syrup instead of honey.

Nutrition Facts:

Calories: 320 | Total Fat: 16g | Saturated Fat: 2g | Cholesterol: 0mg | Sodium: 45mg | Total Carbohydrates: 35g | Dietary Fiber: 8g | Sugars: 7g | Protein: 10g

This quinoa breakfast bowl is an excellent choice for managing type 2 diabetes because it is high in fiber, protein, and healthy fats, which can help regulate blood sugar levels and keep you feeling full and satisfied. The quinoa provides a slow-release of carbohydrates, while the nuts and seeds offer a good source of healthy fats and additional nutrients. This dish can be enjoyed as a nutritious breakfast or a filling snack.

Breakfast Recipes for Blood Sugar Control

11. Scrambled Tofu with Spinach and Tomatoes

Ingredients:
- 1 block (14 oz) firm or extra-firm tofu, crumbled
- 1 tablespoon olive oil
- 1 clove garlic, minced
- 1 cup fresh spinach, chopped
- 1 cup cherry tomatoes, halved
- 1/4 teaspoon turmeric
- 1/4 teaspoon paprika
- Salt and pepper to taste

PreparationTime: 10 minutes
Cook Time: 15 minutes
Total Time: 25 minutes
Serves: 2

Directions:

1. In a large non-stick skillet, heat the olive oil over medium heat.

2. Add the crumbled tofu and garlic to the skillet. Cook, stirring occasionally, for 5-7 minutes, or until the tofu starts to brown.

3. Stir in the chopped spinach and cherry tomatoes. Cook for an additional 3-5 minutes, or until the spinach is wilted and the tomatoes are slightly softened.

4. Season the scrambled tofu mixture with turmeric, paprika, salt, and pepper. Stir to combine.

5. Serve the scrambled tofu warm, either on its own or with a side of whole-grain toast or roasted potatoes.

Storage Instructions:
- Leftover scrambled tofu can be stored in an airtight container in the refrigerator for up to 3 days.

Variations and Tips:
- Add diced onions, bell peppers, or mushrooms for extra flavor and nutrients.
- Use a combination of fresh and frozen spinach for convenience.
- Sprinkle the scrambled tofu with a tablespoon of grated Parmesan cheese or a dollop of plain Greek yogurt for extra creaminess.

Nutrition Facts:
Calories: 180 | Total Fat: 10g | Saturated Fat: 1g | Cholesterol: 0mg | Sodium: 320mg | Total Carbohydrates: 9g | Dietary Fiber: 3g | Sugars: 3g | Protein: 16g

This scrambled tofu dish is an excellent option for managing type 2 diabetes because it is high in protein, low in carbohydrates, and packed with nutrient-dense vegetables. The tofu provides a good source of plant-based protein, while the spinach and tomatoes offer fiber, vitamins, and antioxidants. This dish can be enjoyed as a healthy breakfast, lunch, or dinner.

12. Almond Flour Muffins with Dark Chocolate Chips

Ingredients:
- 2 cups almond flour
- 1/4 cup erythritol or granulated stevia (or 2 tablespoons honey)
- 1 teaspoon baking powder
- 1/4 teaspoon salt
- 3 large eggs
- 1/4 cup unsweetened almond milk
- 2 tablespoons melted coconut oil or unsalted butter
- 1/3 cup dark chocolate chips (at least 70% cacao)

PreparationTime: 10 minutes
Cook Time: 20 minutes
Total Time: 30 minutes
Serves: 12 muffins

Directions:

1. Preheat your oven to 350°F (175°C). Grease a 12-cup muffin tin or line it with paper liners.

2. In a large bowl, whisk together the almond flour, erythritol (or stevia/honey), baking powder, and salt.

3. In a separate bowl, beat the eggs, then stir in the almond milk and melted coconut oil (or butter).

4. Pour the wet ingredients into the dry ingredients and mix until just combined. Fold in the dark chocolate chips.

5. Divide the batter evenly among the prepared muffin cups, filling them about 3/4 full.

6. Bake for 18-20 minutes, or until a toothpick inserted into the center comes out clean.

7. Allow the muffins to cool in the tin for 5 minutes before transferring them to a wire rack to cool completely.

Storage Instructions:
- The muffins can be stored in an airtight container at room temperature for up to 3 days, or in the refrigerator for up to 1 week.

Variations and Tips:
- Use a combination of almond flour and coconut flour for a different texture.
- Swap the dark chocolate chips for chopped nuts, seeds, or dried berries.
- Add a teaspoon of vanilla extract or a pinch of cinnamon for extra flavor.

Nutrition Facts:
Calories: 160 | Total Fat: 13g | Saturated Fat: 5g | Cholesterol: 35mg | Sodium: 105mg | Total Carbohydrates: 8g | Dietary Fiber: 3g | Sugars: 3g | Protein: 5g

13. Whole Wheat English Muffin with Smoked Salmon

Ingredients:
- 1 whole wheat English muffin, toasted
- 2 ounces smoked salmon
- 1 tablespoon cream cheese (or Greek yogurt)
- 1 teaspoon capers (optional)
- 1 tablespoon thinly sliced red onion (optional)
- Freshly ground black pepper to taste

PreparationTime: 5 minutes
Cook Time: 0 minutes
Total Time: 5 minutes
Serves: 1

Directions:

1. Toast the whole wheat English muffin until lightly golden.

2. Spread the cream cheese (or Greek yogurt) evenly over the muffin halves.

3. Top each muffin half with 1 ounce of smoked salmon.

4. If desired, sprinkle the capers and sliced red onion over the salmon.

5. Season with freshly ground black pepper to taste.

Storage Instructions:

- This open-faced sandwich is best enjoyed immediately, as the muffin may become soggy if stored.

Variations and Tips:

- Use a different type of whole-grain bread, such as rye or pumpernickel, instead of an English muffin.
- Add a slice of tomato or a handful of arugula for extra nutrients and flavor.
- For a creamier texture, mix the cream cheese with a bit of lemon juice or dill.

Nutrition Facts:

Calories: 250 | Total Fat: 12g | Saturated Fat: 3g | Cholesterol: 30mg | Sodium: 650mg | Total Carbohydrates: 20g | Dietary Fiber: 4g | Sugars: 3g | Protein: 16g

This whole wheat English muffin with smoked salmon is an excellent option for managing type 2 diabetes. The whole-grain muffin provides a slow release of carbohydrates, while the smoked salmon offers a good source of protein and healthy fats. The cream cheese (or Greek yogurt) adds creaminess and a touch of healthy fat. This open-faced sandwich can be enjoyed as a nutritious breakfast or a light lunch, and the combination of nutrients can help regulate blood sugar levels.

Breakfast Recipes for Blood Sugar Control

14. Buckwheat Pancakes with Raspberries

Ingredients:
- 1 cup buckwheat flour
- 1 teaspoon baking powder
- 1/4 teaspoon baking soda
- 1/4 teaspoon salt
- 1 egg
- 1 cup unsweetened almond milk
- 1 tablespoon honey (optional)
- 1 cup fresh raspberries

PreparationTime: 10 minutes
Cook Time: 15 minutes
Total Time: 25 minutes
Serves: 2 (3 pancakes per serving)

Directions:
1. In a medium bowl, whisk together the buckwheat flour, baking powder, baking soda, and salt.

2. In a separate bowl, beat the egg, then stir in the almond milk and honey (if using).

3. Pour the wet ingredients into the dry ingredients and stir just until combined (do not overmix).

4. Heat a non-stick skillet or griddle over medium heat. Scoop about 1/4 cup of the batter onto the hot surface and cook for 2-3 minutes, or until bubbles start to form on the surface.

5. Flip the pancake and cook for another 2-3 minutes, or until golden brown.

6. Repeat with the remaining batter, making about 6 pancakes total.

7. Serve the buckwheat pancakes warm, topped with the fresh raspberries.

Storage Instructions:
- Leftover pancakes can be stored in an airtight container in the refrigerator for up to 3 days, or frozen for up to 3 months.

Variations and Tips:
- Use a combination of buckwheat and whole wheat flour for a heartier texture.
- Add a sprinkle of cinnamon or a tablespoon of chopped nuts for extra flavor.
- Serve the pancakes with a side of Greek yogurt or a drizzle of nut butter for additional protein.

Nutrition Facts:
Calories: 240 | Total Fat: 5g | Saturated Fat: 1g | Cholesterol: 55mg | Sodium: 390mg | Total Carbohydrates: 40g | Dietary Fiber: 6g | Sugars: 10g | Protein: 9g

These buckwheat pancakes are an excellent choice for managing type 2 diabetes. Buckwheat is a gluten-free, high-fiber grain that can help regulate blood sugar levels. The raspberries provide a natural sweetness and a boost of antioxidants. This dish is a nutritious and satisfying breakfast option that can help keep your blood sugar in check.

Breakfast Recipes for Blood Sugar Control

15. Peanut Butter and Banana Smoothie

Ingredients:
- 1 medium ripe banana, frozen
- 2 tablespoons natural peanut butter
- 1 cup unsweetened almond milk
- 1 tablespoon ground flaxseed
- 1/2 teaspoon vanilla extract (optional)

PreparationTime: 5 minutes
Cook Time: 0 minutes
Total Time: 5 minutes
Serves: 1

Directions:

1. In a high-speed blender, combine the frozen banana, peanut butter, almond milk, ground flaxseed, and vanilla extract (if using).

2. Blend the ingredients until smooth and creamy.

3. Pour the smoothie into a glass and enjoy immediately.

Storage Instructions:- This smoothie is best enjoyed immediately, as the banana and peanut butter may not keep well if stored.

Variations and Tips:

- Use any type of nut butter, such as almond butter or cashew butter, instead of peanut butter.

- Add a handful of spinach or kale for extra nutrients.

- Sprinkle a tablespoon of unsweetened coconut flakes or a dash of cinnamon on top for extra flavor.

- For a thicker consistency, use less almond milk or add a few ice cubes.

Nutrition Facts:

Calories: 320 | Total Fat: 18g | Saturated Fat: 3g | Cholesterol: 0mg | Sodium: 160mg | Total Carbohydrates: 32g | Dietary Fiber: 6g | Sugars: 14g | Protein: 12g

This peanut butter and banana smoothie is an excellent choice for managing type 2 diabetes. The combination of the banana, peanut butter, and almond milk provides a good balance of carbohydrates, protein, and healthy fats to help regulate blood sugar levels. The ground flaxseed adds fiber and omega-3 fatty acids, which can also be beneficial for diabetes management. This smoothie can be enjoyed as a nutritious breakfast or a satisfying snack.

16. Egg White Frittata with Zucchini and Cheese

Ingredients:
- 8 large egg whites
- 1/4 cup unsweetened almond milk
- 1/4 teaspoon salt
- 1/4 teaspoon black pepper
- 1 cup diced zucchini
- 1/2 cup shredded low-fat cheddar cheese
- 1 tablespoon chopped fresh basil (optional)

PreparationTime: 10 minutes
Cook Time: 20 minutes
Total Time: 30 minutes
Serves: 4

Directions:

1. Preheat your oven to 375°F (190°C). Grease a 9-inch pie dish or oven-safe skillet with non-stick cooking spray.

2. In a medium bowl, whisk together the egg whites, almond milk, salt, and black pepper until well combined.

3. Stir in the diced zucchini and shredded cheddar cheese.

4. Pour the egg mixture into the prepared pie dish or skillet.

5. Bake for 18-20 minutes, or until the frittata is set and lightly golden on top.

6. Remove the frittata from the oven and let it cool for 5 minutes.

7. Slice the frittata and serve warm, garnished with the chopped fresh basil (if using).

Storage Instructions:
- Leftover frittata can be stored in an airtight container in the refrigerator for up to 3 days.

Variations and Tips:
- Use a combination of whole eggs and egg whites for a richer texture.
- Swap the zucchini for other vegetables, such as spinach, bell peppers, or onions.
- Try different types of cheese, such as feta or goat cheese, for a variety of flavors.
- Serve the frittata with a side of roasted tomatoes or a fresh salad for a complete meal.

Nutrition Facts:
Calories: 120 | Total Fat: 5g | Saturated Fat: 2g | Cholesterol: 10mg | Sodium: 320mg | Total Carbohydrates: 4g | Dietary Fiber: 1g | Sugars: 2g | Protein: 14g

This egg white frittata is an excellent choice for managing type 2 diabetes. The egg whites provide a good source of protein, while the zucchini and low-fat cheese add fiber, vitamins, and healthy fats. The almond milk helps keep the frittata moist and creamy without adding too many carbohydrates. This dish can be enjoyed as a nutritious breakfast, lunch, or dinner.

Breakfast Recipes for Blood Sugar Control

17. Breakfast Burrito with Black Beans and Salsa

Ingredients:
- 2 whole wheat tortillas
- 1/2 cup canned black beans, rinsed and drained
- 2 eggs, scrambled
- 1/4 cup diced bell pepper
- 2 tablespoons diced onion
- 2 tablespoons salsa
- 1 tablespoon shredded low-fat cheddar cheese
- Salt and pepper to taste

PreparationTime: 10 minutes
Cook Time: 15 minutes
Total Time: 25 minutes
Serves: 2

Directions:

1. In a small skillet, sauté the diced bell pepper and onion over medium heat until softened, about 5 minutes.

2. In a separate bowl, scramble the eggs until cooked through.

3. In the center of each whole wheat tortilla, layer the scrambled eggs, black beans, sautéed vegetables, salsa, and shredded cheese.

4. Fold the bottom of the tortilla up, then fold in the sides and continue rolling to create a burrito.

5. Serve the breakfast burritos warm.

Storage Instructions:
- Leftover burritos can be wrapped individually in foil or parchment paper and stored in the refrigerator for up to 3 days.

Variations and Tips:
- Use a combination of eggs and egg whites for a lower-calorie option.
- Add diced avocado or a sprinkle of chopped cilantro for extra flavor and nutrients.
- For a spicier version, use a hotter salsa or add a pinch of cayenne pepper.
- Serve the burritos with a side of plain Greek yogurt or a small green salad.

Nutrition Facts:
Calories: 300 | Total Fat: 10g | Saturated Fat: 3g | Cholesterol: 185mg | Sodium: 650mg | Total Carbohydrates: 35g | Dietary Fiber: 8g | Sugars: 3g | Protein: 16g

This breakfast burrito is an excellent choice for managing type 2 diabetes. The whole wheat tortilla provides complex carbohydrates, the black beans offer fiber and protein, and the eggs and cheese add a good source of healthy fats and protein. The salsa and vegetables provide additional nutrients and antioxidants. This dish can be enjoyed as a satisfying and balanced breakfast or brunch.

Breakfast Recipes for Blood Sugar Control

18. Steel-Cut Oats with Apple Slices and Walnuts

Ingredients:
- 1/2 cup steel-cut oats
- 1 cup unsweetened almond milk
- 1/2 cup water
- 1 medium apple, cored and sliced
- 2 tablespoons chopped walnuts
- 1 teaspoon ground cinnamon
- 1 tablespoon honey (optional)

PreparationTime: 5 minutes
Cook Time: 20 minutes
Total Time: 25 minutes
Serves: 2

Directions:

1. In a medium saucepan, combine the steel-cut oats, almond milk, and water. Bring the mixture to a boil over medium-high heat.

2. Once boiling, reduce the heat to low and let the oats simmer, stirring occasionally, for 18-20 minutes, or until the oats are tender and the mixture has thickened.

3. Remove the saucepan from the heat and stir in the sliced apple, chopped walnuts, and ground cinnamon.

4. If desired, drizzle the honey over the top of the oatmeal.

5. Serve the steel-cut oats warm.

Storage Instructions:
- Leftover oatmeal can be stored in an airtight container in the refrigerator for up to 4 days. Reheat before serving.

Variations and Tips:
- Use a different type of nut, such as pecans or almonds, instead of walnuts.
- Add a spoonful of peanut butter or almond butter for extra protein and flavor.
- Top the oatmeal with fresh berries or a sprinkle of unsweetened coconut flakes.

Nutrition Facts:
Calories: 280 | Total Fat: 12g | Saturated Fat: 1g | Cholesterol: 0mg | Sodium: 45mg | Total Carbohydrates: 38g | Dietary Fiber: 7g | Sugars: 12g | Protein: 8g

This steel-cut oats dish is an excellent choice for managing type 2 diabetes. Steel-cut oats are a whole grain that provides a slow release of carbohydrates, helping to regulate blood sugar levels. The addition of apples, walnuts, and cinnamon provides fiber, healthy fats, and antioxidants, which can also be beneficial for diabetes management. This breakfast can be enjoyed as a nutritious and satisfying start to the day.

19. Green Smoothie with Kale, Pineapple, and Coconut Water

Ingredients:
- 1 cup fresh kale, stems removed
- 1 cup frozen pineapple chunks
- 1 cup unsweetened coconut water
- 1 tablespoon chia seeds
- 1 tablespoon ground flaxseed
- 1/2 inch fresh ginger, peeled (optional)

PreparationTime: 5 minutes
Cook Time: 0 minutes
Total Time: 5 minutes
Serves: 1

Directions:

1. In a high-speed blender, combine the kale, frozen pineapple, coconut water, chia seeds, flaxseed, and ginger (if using).

2. Blend the ingredients until smooth and creamy.

3. Pour the green smoothie into a glass and enjoy immediately.

Storage Instructions:
- This smoothie is best enjoyed immediately, as the kale and pineapple may not keep well if stored.

Variations and Tips:
- Use a combination of kale and spinach for a different flavor profile.

- Add a scoop of protein powder or a tablespoon of almond butter for extra protein.

- Substitute the pineapple with other frozen fruits, such as mango or berries.

- For a creamier texture, use unsweetened almond milk or Greek yogurt instead of coconut water.

Nutrition Facts:
Calories: 200 | Total Fat: 7g | Saturated Fat: 1g | Cholesterol: 0mg | Sodium: 120mg | Total Carbohydrates: 28g | Dietary Fiber: 7g | Sugars: 15g | Protein: 6g

This green smoothie is an excellent choice for managing type 2 diabetes. The kale provides a nutrient-dense base, while the pineapple and coconut water add natural sweetness and hydration. The chia seeds and flaxseed offer a good source of fiber, healthy fats, and antioxidants, which can help regulate blood sugar levels and support overall health. This smoothie can be enjoyed as a nutritious breakfast or a refreshing snack.

20. Breakfast Quinoa with Cinnamon and Apples

Ingredients:
- 1 cup cooked quinoa
- 1 cup unsweetened almond milk
- 1 medium apple, diced
- 1 teaspoon ground cinnamon
- 1 tablespoon chopped walnuts (optional)
- 1 teaspoon honey (optional)

PreparationTime: 5 minutes
Cook Time: 15 minutes
Total Time: 20 minutes
Serves: 2

Directions:

1. In a small saucepan, combine the cooked quinoa and almond milk. Heat over medium heat, stirring occasionally, until the mixture is warm and creamy, about 5 minutes.

2. Remove the saucepan from the heat and stir in the diced apple and ground cinnamon.

3. Divide the quinoa mixture between two bowls.

4. If desired, top each serving with chopped walnuts and a drizzle of honey.

Storage Instructions:

- Leftover quinoa can be stored in an airtight container in the refrigerator for up to 4 days.

Variations and Tips:

- Use a different type of milk, such as cow's milk or coconut milk, instead of almond milk.

- Add a spoonful of nut butter or a sprinkle of shredded coconut for extra flavor and texture.

- Swap the apples for other diced fruit, such as pears or berries.

- For a creamier texture, mash half of the apple into the quinoa before serving.

Nutrition Facts:

Calories: 240 | Total Fat: 7g | Saturated Fat: 1g | Cholesterol: 0mg | Sodium: 45mg | Total Carbohydrates: 37g | Dietary Fiber: 6g | Sugars: 12g | Protein: 8g

This breakfast quinoa dish is an excellent choice for managing type 2 diabetes. Quinoa is a high-fiber, high-protein grain that can help regulate blood sugar levels. The addition of apples, cinnamon, and walnuts (if using) provides a good source of fiber, antioxidants, and healthy fats, which can also be beneficial for diabetes management. This dish can be enjoyed as a nutritious and satisfying breakfast or a filling snack.

Breakfast Recipes for Blood Sugar Control

21. Grilled Chicken Salad with Mixed Greens and Avocado

PreparationTime: 10 minutes
Cook Time: 10 minutes
Total Time: 20 minutes
Serves: 2

Ingredients:
- 2 boneless, skinless chicken breasts
- 1 tablespoon olive oil
- 1/4 teaspoon salt
- 1/4 teaspoon black pepper
- 4 cups mixed greens (such as spinach, arugula, and kale)
- 1 avocado, sliced
- 1/4 cup cherry tomatoes, halved
- 2 tablespoons balsamic vinaigrette (or your preferred dressing)

Directions:
1. Preheat your grill or grill pan to medium-high heat.
2. Brush the chicken breasts with the olive oil and season with salt and pepper.
3. Grill the chicken for 5-7 minutes per side, or until it's cooked through and reaches an internal temperature of 165°F (74°C).
4. Remove the chicken from the grill and let it rest for 5 minutes before slicing it into strips.
5. In a large salad bowl, combine the mixed greens, sliced avocado, and cherry tomatoes.
6. Top the salad with the grilled chicken strips and drizzle the balsamic vinaigrette over the top.
7. Serve the salad immediately.

Storage Instructions:
- The grilled chicken can be stored in an airtight container in the refrigerator for up to 3 days.
- The salad ingredients can be stored separately in the refrigerator for up to 3 days.

Variations and Tips:
- Use a different type of protein, such as grilled salmon or roasted tofu, instead of chicken.
- Add other vegetables, such as cucumber, bell peppers, or roasted sweet potatoes, to the salad.
- Try different types of dressings, such as a lemon-garlic vinaigrette or a creamy avocado dressing.
- For a heartier meal, serve the salad with a side of whole-grain crackers or a slice of whole-wheat bread.

Nutrition Facts:
Calories: 350 | Total Fat: 18g | Saturated Fat: 3g | Cholesterol: 70mg | Sodium: 450mg | Total Carbohydrates: 16g | Dietary Fiber: 9g | Sugars: 4g | Protein: 34g

This grilled chicken salad is an excellent choice for managing type 2 diabetes. The combination of lean protein, healthy fats, and fiber-rich greens and vegetables can help regulate blood sugar levels and keep you feeling full and satisfied. The avocado provides additional healthy fats, while the balsamic vinaigrette adds flavor without too many added sugars. This dish can be enjoyed as a nutritious lunch or dinner.

22. Lentil Soup with Carrots and Celery

Ingredients:
- 1 tablespoon olive oil
- 1 onion, diced
- 3 cloves garlic, minced
- 2 carrots, peeled and diced
- 2 stalks celery, diced
- 1 cup dried brown or green lentils, rinsed
- 4 cups low-sodium vegetable or chicken broth
- 1 (14.5 oz) can diced tomatoes
- 1 teaspoon dried thyme
- 1/2 teaspoon ground cumin
- Salt and pepper to taste
- Chopped parsley for garnish (optional)

PreparationTime: 15 minutes
Cook Time: 45 minutes
Total Time: 1 hour
Serves: 4

Directions:
1. In a large pot or Dutch oven, heat the olive oil over medium heat.
2. Add the diced onion and sauté for 3-4 minutes, until translucent.
3. Add the minced garlic, diced carrots, and diced celery. Sauté for an additional 5 minutes.
4. Stir in the rinsed lentils, vegetable or chicken broth, diced tomatoes, dried thyme, and ground cumin.
5. Bring the soup to a boil, then reduce the heat and let it simmer for 35-40 minutes, or until the lentils are tender.
6. Season the soup with salt and pepper to taste.
7. Serve the lentil soup hot, garnished with chopped parsley if desired.

Storage Instructions:
- Leftover lentil soup can be stored in an airtight container in the refrigerator for up to 4 days or in the freezer for up to 3 months.

Variations and Tips:
- Add diced potatoes or sweet potatoes for extra heartiness.
- Use a combination of broth and water to reduce the sodium content.
- Stir in a handful of spinach or kale towards the end of cooking for added nutrients.
- Serve the soup with a side of whole-grain crackers or a slice of whole-wheat bread.

Nutrition Facts:
Calories: 250 | Total Fat: 5g | Saturated Fat: 1g | Cholesterol: 0mg | Sodium: 450mg | Total Carbohydrates: 38g | Dietary Fiber: 12g | Sugars: 8g | Protein: 15g

This lentil soup is an excellent choice for managing type 2 diabetes. Lentils are a high-fiber, high-protein legume that can help regulate blood sugar levels. The addition of carrots, celery, and tomatoes provides a variety of vitamins, minerals, and antioxidants. This soup is a nutritious and filling meal that can be enjoyed for lunch or dinner.

Lunch Recipes for Sustained Energy

23. Turkey and Spinach Wrap

Ingredients:
- 1 whole-wheat tortilla or wrap
- 2-3 ounces sliced turkey breast
- 1/2 cup fresh spinach leaves
- 1 tablespoon hummus
- 1 tablespoon sliced cucumber
- 1 tablespoon shredded carrots
- 1 teaspoon olive oil (optional)
- Salt and pepper to taste

PreparationTime: 10 minutes
Cook Time: 0 minutes
Total Time: 10 minutes
Serves: 1

Directions:

1. Lay the whole-wheat tortilla or wrap on a flat surface.

2. Spread the hummus evenly over the center of the tortilla.

3. Layer the sliced turkey, fresh spinach leaves, sliced cucumber, and shredded carrots on top of

the hummus.

4. If desired, drizzle the olive oil over the filling.

5. Season with salt and pepper to taste.

6. Fold the bottom of the tortilla up, then fold in the sides and continue rolling to create a wrap.

7. Serve the turkey and spinach wrap immediately.

Storage Instructions:
- Wrapped sandwiches can be stored in an airtight container in the refrigerator for up to 3 days.

Variations and Tips:
- Use a different type of protein, such as grilled chicken or roasted tofu, instead of turkey.
- Add other vegetables, such as bell peppers, avocado, or sprouts, to the wrap.
- Try different types of spreads, such as cream cheese or pesto, instead of hummus.
- For a heartier meal, serve the wrap with a side of fresh fruit or a small salad.

Nutrition Facts:
Calories: 280 | Total Fat: 9g | Saturated Fat: 1g | Cholesterol: 30mg | Sodium: 650mg | Total
Carbohydrates: 30g | Dietary Fiber: 6g | Sugars: 3g | Protein: 20g

This turkey and spinach wrap is an excellent choice for managing type 2 diabetes. The whole-wheat tortilla provides complex carbohydrates, while the turkey and hummus offer a good source of protein. The spinach, cucumber, and carrots add fiber, vitamins, and antioxidants. This wrap can be enjoyed as a quick and nutritious lunch or a satisfying snack.

Lunch Recipes for Sustained Energy

24. Quinoa Salad with Chickpeas and Feta

Ingredients:
- 1 cup uncooked quinoa, rinsed
- 2 cups low-sodium vegetable or chicken broth
- 1 (15 oz) can chickpeas, rinsed and drained
- 1 cup diced cucumber
- 1/2 cup crumbled feta cheese
- 1/4 cup chopped fresh parsley
- 2 tablespoons olive oil
- 2 tablespoons lemon juice
- 1 teaspoon Dijon mustard
- 1/4 teaspoon salt
- 1/4 teaspoon black pepper

PreparationTime: 15 minutes
Cook Time: 15 minutes
Total Time: 30 minutes
Serves: 4

Directions:
1. In a medium saucepan, combine the rinsed quinoa and broth. Bring the mixture to a boil, then reduce the heat, cover, and simmer for 15 minutes, or until the quinoa is tender and the liquid is absorbed.
2. Transfer the cooked quinoa to a large bowl and let it cool slightly.
3. Add the rinsed and drained chickpeas, diced cucumber, crumbled feta cheese, and chopped parsley to the bowl with the quinoa.
4. In a small bowl, whisk together the olive oil, lemon juice, Dijon mustard, salt, and black pepper.
5. Pour the dressing over the quinoa salad and toss gently to combine.
6. Serve the quinoa salad chilled or at room temperature.

Storage Instructions:
- The quinoa salad can be stored in an airtight container in the refrigerator for up to 4 days.

Variations and Tips:
- Use a different type of bean, such as black beans or edamame, instead of chickpeas.
- Add diced tomatoes, bell peppers, or red onion for extra flavor and color.
- Swap the feta cheese for another type of crumbled cheese, such as goat cheese or cotija.
- Serve the quinoa salad on a bed of mixed greens for a more substantial meal.

Nutrition Facts:
Calories: 320 | Total Fat: 13g | Saturated Fat: 3g | Cholesterol: 15mg | Sodium: 450mg | Total Carbohydrates: 38g | Dietary Fiber: 8g | Sugars: 3g | Protein: 12g

This quinoa salad with chickpeas and feta is an excellent choice for managing type 2 diabetes. Quinoa is a high-fiber, high-protein grain that can help regulate blood sugar levels, while the chickpeas and feta provide additional protein and healthy fats. The vegetables and herbs add a variety of vitamins, minerals, and antioxidants. This salad can be enjoyed as a nutritious lunch or a light dinner.

Lunch Recipes for Sustained Energy

25. Vegetable Stir-Fry with Tofu and Brown Rice

Ingredients:
- 1 cup uncooked brown rice
- 1 block (14 oz) extra-firm tofu, drained and cubed
- 2 tablespoons sesame oil, divided
- 2 cloves garlic, minced
- 1 inch piece fresh ginger, peeled and grated
- 1 red bell pepper, sliced
- 1 cup broccoli florets
- 1 cup sliced mushrooms
- 1 cup snow peas or snap peas
- 2 tablespoons low-sodium soy sauce
- 1 tablespoon rice vinegar
- 1 teaspoon sesame seeds (optional)

PreparationTime: 20 minutes
Cook Time: 30 minutes
Total Time: 50 minutes
Serves: 4

Directions:
1. Cook the brown rice according to package instructions.
2. In a large skillet or wok, heat 1 tablespoon of sesame oil over medium-high heat. Add the cubed tofu and cook, stirring occasionally, until lightly browned on all sides, about 5-7 minutes. Transfer the tofu to a plate and set aside.
3. In the same skillet, heat the remaining 1 tablespoon of sesame oil. Add the garlic and ginger and cook for 1 minute, stirring constantly, until fragrant.
4. Add the bell pepper, broccoli, mushrooms, and snow peas. Stir-fry for 5-7 minutes, or until the vegetables are tender-crisp.
5. Return the cooked tofu to the skillet and add the soy sauce and rice vinegar. Toss everything together and cook for an additional 2-3 minutes.
6. Serve the stir-fry over the cooked brown rice and sprinkle with sesame seeds, if desired.

Storage Instructions:
Leftovers can be stored in an airtight container in the refrigerator for up to 4 days.

Variations and Tips:
- Use a variety of vegetables, such as carrots, zucchini, or bok choy, to change up the flavors.
- Add a splash of hot sauce or chili oil for a spicier version.
- Swap the tofu for chicken or shrimp for a different protein option.
- Serve with steamed edamame or a side salad for a more complete meal.

Nutrition Facts:

Calories: 320 - Total Fat: 14g - Saturated Fat: 2g - Cholesterol: 0mg - Sodium: 420mg
Total Carbohydrates: 37g - Dietary Fiber: 6g - Total Sugars: 4g -Protein: 16g

Lunch Recipes for Sustained Energy

26. Tuna Salad with Olive Oil and Lemon Dressing

Ingredients:
- 2 (5 oz) cans tuna, drained
- 1/2 cup diced celery
- 1/4 cup diced red onion
- 2 tablespoons chopped fresh parsley
- 2 tablespoons olive oil
- 2 tablespoons lemon juice
- 1 teaspoon Dijon mustard
- Salt and black pepper to taste

PreparationTime: 15 minutes
Cook Time: 0 minutes
Total Time: 15 minutes

Serves: 4

Directions:

1. In a medium bowl, combine the drained tuna, celery, red onion, and parsley.

2. In a small bowl, whisk together the olive oil, lemon juice, and Dijon mustard.

3. Pour the dressing over the tuna mixture and gently toss to coat.

4. Season with salt and black pepper to taste.

5. Serve the tuna salad on a bed of greens, in a sandwich, or with crackers.

Storage Instructions:

The tuna salad can be stored in an airtight container in the refrigerator for up to 3 days.

Variations and Tips:

- Add diced cucumber or cherry tomatoes for extra crunch and flavor.
- Use Greek yogurt instead of olive oil for a creamy dressing.
- Sprinkle with chopped walnuts or sliced almonds for added texture.
- Serve the tuna salad stuffed in avocado halves or tomato cups.

Nutrition Facts:

Calories: 160 - Total Fat: 10g - Saturated Fat: 1.5g - Cholesterol: 30mg
Sodium: 360mg - Total Carbohydrates: 3g - Dietary Fiber: 1g - Total Sugars: 1g - Protein: 15g

Lunch Recipes for Sustained Energy

27. Roasted Beet and Goat Cheese Salad

Ingredients:
- 3 medium beets, peeled and cut into 1-inch cubes
- 2 tablespoons olive oil
- Salt and black pepper to taste
- 4 cups mixed greens
- 1/2 cup crumbled goat cheese
- 2 tablespoons toasted walnuts
- 2 tablespoons balsamic vinegar
- 1 tablespoon Dijon mustard
- 1 tablespoon honey

PreparationTime: 20 minutes
Cook Time: 45 minutes
Total Time: 1 hour 5 minutes
Serves: 4

Directions:
1. Preheat the oven to 400°F (200°C).
2. Toss the cubed beets with 1 tablespoon of olive oil and season with salt and black pepper.
3. Spread the beets on a baking sheet and roast for 35-45 minutes, or until tender and lightly caramelized, stirring halfway through.
4. In a small bowl, whisk together the remaining 1 tablespoon of olive oil, balsamic vinegar, Dijon mustard, and honey to make the dressing.
5. In a large salad bowl, combine the mixed greens, roasted beets, crumbled goat cheese, and toasted walnuts.
6. Drizzle the dressing over the salad and toss gently to coat.

Storage Instructions:
The roasted beets can be stored in an airtight container in the refrigerator for up to 5 days. The salad can be assembled and dressed just before serving.

Variations and Tips:
- Use a variety of beets, such as golden or rainbow beets, for a more colorful salad.
- Add sliced avocado or grilled chicken for a more substantial meal.
- Substitute feta cheese or blue cheese for the goat cheese, if desired.
- Sprinkle with chopped fresh herbs, such as basil or dill, for extra flavor.

Nutrition Facts:

Calories: 190 - Total Fat: 12g - Saturated Fat: 4g - Cholesterol: 15mg
Sodium: 320mg - Total Carbohydrates: 16g - Dietary Fiber: 4g - Total Sugars: 10g - Protein: 8g

This salad is a great option for managing type 2 diabetes. The beets are a low-glycemic vegetable, the goat cheese provides healthy fats, and the greens are a nutrient-dense source of fiber. The dressing is made with a small amount of honey, which can help satisfy a sweet craving without spiking blood sugar levels.

28. Grilled Salmon with Asparagus

Ingredients:
- 4 (6 oz) salmon fillets
- 1 lb asparagus, trimmed
- 2 tablespoons olive oil, divided
- 1 tablespoon lemon juice
- 1 teaspoon Dijon mustard
- 1 clove garlic, minced
- Salt and black pepper to taste

Preparation Time: 15 minutes
Cook Time: 20 minutes
Total Time: 35 minutes
Serves: 4

Directions:
1. Preheat grill or grill pan to medium-high heat.

2. In a small bowl, whisk together 1 tablespoon of olive oil, lemon juice, Dijon mustard, and garlic. Season with salt and black pepper.

3. Toss the asparagus with the remaining 1 tablespoon of olive oil and season with salt and black pepper.

4. Grill the salmon fillets for 4-6 minutes per side, or until cooked through and flaky.

5. Grill the asparagus for 5-7 minutes, turning occasionally, until tender-crisp.

6. Drizzle the lemon-Dijon dressing over the grilled salmon and asparagus.

Storage Instructions:
Leftovers can be stored in an airtight container in the refrigerator for up to 3 days.

Variations and Tips:
- Use a different type of fish, such as halibut or cod, if desired.
- Add sliced lemon or fresh herbs, like dill or parsley, for extra flavor.
- Serve the salmon and asparagus over a bed of mixed greens or quinoa for a more substantial meal.
- For a creamier dressing, substitute Greek yogurt for the Dijon mustard.

Nutrition Facts:

Calories: 260 - Total Fat: 14g - Saturated Fat: 2.5g - Cholesterol: 70mg - Sodium: 320mg
Total Carbohydrates: 6g - Dietary Fiber: 3g - Total Sugars: 2g - Protein: 28g

This grilled salmon and asparagus dish is an excellent choice for managing type 2 diabetes. Salmon is a rich source of omega-3 fatty acids, which can help improve insulin sensitivity and reduce inflammation. Asparagus is a low-carb, high-fiber vegetable that can help regulate blood sugar levels. The simple lemon-Dijon dressing provides flavor without added sugars.

Lunch Recipes for Sustained Energy

29. Black Bean and Corn Salad with Cilantro

Ingredients:
- 1 (15 oz) can black beans, rinsed and drained
- 1 (15 oz) can corn, drained
- 1 red bell pepper, diced
- 1/2 red onion, diced
- 1/4 cup chopped fresh cilantro
- 2 tablespoons olive oil
- 2 tablespoons lime juice
- 1 teaspoon ground cumin
- 1/4 teaspoon chili powder
- Salt and black pepper to taste

PreparationTime: 20 minutes
Cook Time: 0 minutes
Total Time: 20 minutes
Serves: 6

Directions:

1. In a large bowl, combine the rinsed and drained black beans, drained corn, diced red bell pepper, diced red onion, and chopped fresh cilantro.

2. In a small bowl, whisk together the olive oil, lime juice, ground cumin, and chili powder.

3. Pour the dressing over the black bean and corn salad and toss gently to coat.

4. Season with salt and black pepper to taste.

5. Serve chilled or at room temperature.

Storage Instructions:
The salad can be stored in an airtight container in the refrigerator for up to 4 days.

Variations and Tips:
- Add diced avocado or cherry tomatoes for extra flavor and nutrients.
- Substitute feta or queso fresco cheese for a creamy texture.
- Use a combination of bell peppers (red, yellow, and orange) for a more colorful salad.
- Serve the salad on a bed of mixed greens or with baked tortilla chips.

Nutrition Facts:

Calories: 160 - Total Fat: 6g - Saturated Fat: 1g - Cholesterol: 0mg
Sodium: 320mg - Total Carbohydrates: 22g - Dietary Fiber: 6g - Total Sugars: 4g - Protein: 6g

This black bean and corn salad is an excellent choice for managing type 2 diabetes. The combination of fiber-rich black beans and low-glycemic corn helps to regulate blood sugar levels. The fresh cilantro, lime juice, and spices add flavor without the need for added sugars or unhealthy fats. This salad can be enjoyed as a side dish or a light main course.

Lunch Recipes for Sustained Energy

30. Spinach and Strawberry Salad with Balsamic Vinaigrette

Ingredients:
- 5 oz baby spinach
- 1 cup fresh strawberries, sliced
- 1/4 cup crumbled feta cheese
- 2 tablespoons sliced almonds
- 2 tablespoons balsamic vinegar
- 1 tablespoon olive oil
- 1 teaspoon Dijon mustard
- 1 teaspoon honey
- Salt and black pepper to taste

PreparationTime: 15 minutes
Cook Time: 0 minutes
Total Time: 15 minutes
Serves: 4

Directions:
1. In a large salad bowl, combine the baby spinach, sliced strawberries, crumbled feta cheese, and sliced almonds.

2. In a small bowl, whisk together the balsamic vinegar, olive oil, Dijon mustard, and honey. Season with salt and black pepper to taste.

3. Drizzle the balsamic vinaigrette over the salad and toss gently to coat.

Storage Instructions:
The salad can be assembled and stored in the refrigerator for up to 2 days, but the dressing should be added just before serving to prevent the spinach from wilting.

Variations and Tips:
- Use a mix of greens, such as arugula or kale, in addition to the spinach.
- Add grilled chicken or shrimp for a more substantial meal.
- Substitute goat cheese or blue cheese for the feta cheese.
- Use different types of nuts, such as pecans or walnuts, for variety.
- Experiment with different fruit, such as blueberries or mandarin oranges.

Nutrition Facts:

Calories: 140 - Total Fat: 9g - Saturated Fat: 2g - Cholesterol: 10mg
Sodium: 260mg - Total Carbohydrates: 12g - Dietary Fiber: 3g - Total Sugars: 7g - Protein: 5g

This spinach and strawberry salad is an excellent choice for managing type 2 diabetes. The spinach is a nutrient-dense green that is low in carbohydrates, while the strawberries provide a sweet and low-glycemic fruit. The balsamic vinaigrette dressing is made with a small amount of honey, which can help satisfy a sweet craving without spiking blood sugar levels. The feta cheese and almonds provide healthy fats and protein to help keep you feeling full and satisfied.

Lunch Recipes for Sustained Energy

31. Greek Salad with Chicken

Ingredients:

PreparationTime: 20 minutes
Cook Time: 15 minutes
Total Time: 35 minutes
Serves: 4

- 1 lb boneless, skinless chicken breasts
- 1 tablespoon olive oil
- 1 teaspoon dried oregano
- Salt and black pepper to taste
- 6 cups chopped romaine lettuce
- 1 cup cherry tomatoes, halved
- 1/2 cup diced cucumber
- 1/4 cup sliced red onion
- 1/4 cup pitted kalamata olives, halved
- 1/4 cup crumbled feta cheese
- 2 tablespoons lemon juice
- 1 tablespoon red wine vinegar
- 1 tablespoon olive oil
- 1 teaspoon Dijon mustard
- 1 clove garlic, minced
- Salt and black pepper to taste

Directions:

1. Preheat the oven to 400°F (200°C).
2. Season the chicken breasts with the dried oregano, salt, and black pepper.
3. Heat 1 tablespoon of olive oil in a skillet over medium-high heat. Add the chicken and cook for 6-8 minutes per side, or until cooked through. Let the chicken rest for 5 minutes, then slice or chop it.
4. In a large salad bowl, combine the chopped romaine lettuce, cherry tomatoes, diced cucumber, sliced red onion, and halved kalamata olives.
5. In a small bowl, whisk together the lemon juice, red wine vinegar, 1 tablespoon of olive oil, Dijon mustard, and minced garlic. Season with salt and black pepper to taste.
6. Add the sliced or chopped chicken to the salad and drizzle the dressing over the top. Toss gently to coat.
7. Sprinkle the crumbled feta cheese over the salad before serving.

Storage Instructions:

The salad can be assembled and stored in the refrigerator for up to 2 days, but the dressing should be added just before serving.

Variations and Tips:

- Use grilled or roasted salmon or shrimp instead of chicken for a different protein option.
- Add diced bell peppers or sliced radishes for extra crunch and color.
- Substitute crumbled goat cheese or shredded mozzarella for the feta cheese.
- Serve the salad with a side of whole-grain pita bread or quinoa for a more substantial meal.

Lunch Recipes for Sustained Energy

32. Roasted Vegetable and Hummus Wrap

Ingredients:
- 1 medium zucchini, sliced
- 1 red bell pepper, sliced
- 1 cup sliced mushrooms
- 1 tablespoon olive oil
- Salt and black pepper to taste
- 4 (8-inch) whole-wheat tortillas
- 1/2 cup hummus
- 1 cup baby spinach leaves
- 1/4 cup crumbled feta cheese

PreparationTime: 20 minutes
Cook Time: 25 minutes
Total Time: 45 minutes
Serves: 4

Directions:
1. Preheat the oven to 400°F (200°C).
2. In a large bowl, toss the sliced zucchini, red bell pepper, and mushrooms with the olive oil. Season with salt and black pepper.
3. Spread the vegetables on a baking sheet and roast for 20-25 minutes, or until tender and lightly browned, stirring halfway through.
4. Spread 2 tablespoons of hummus onto each whole-wheat tortilla.
5. Top the hummus with the roasted vegetables, baby spinach leaves, and crumbled feta cheese.
6. Fold the sides of the tortilla in and then roll it up tightly to create a wrap.

Storage Instructions:
The roasted vegetables can be stored in an airtight container in the refrigerator for up to 4 days. Assemble the wraps just before serving for the best texture.

Variations and Tips:
- Use a variety of roasted vegetables, such as eggplant, carrots, or onions.
- Add grilled or roasted chicken or turkey for extra protein.
- Substitute other types of cheese, such as goat cheese or shredded cheddar.
- Use a flavored hummus, such as roasted red pepper or garlic, for added flavor.
- Serve the wraps with a side of fresh fruit or a small salad for a more complete meal.

Nutrition Facts:

Calories: 320 - Total Fat: 14g - Saturated Fat: 3g - Cholesterol: 10mg - Sodium: 650mg
Total Carbohydrates: 38g - Dietary Fiber: 7g - Total Sugars: 5g - Protein: 12g

This roasted vegetable and hummus wrap is an excellent choice for managing type 2 diabetes. The whole-wheat tortilla provides complex carbohydrates and fiber, while the hummus and roasted vegetables offer a nutrient-dense and low-glycemic combination. The feta cheese adds a creamy texture and a boost of protein. This wrap can be enjoyed as a satisfying lunch or light dinner.

Lunch Recipes for Sustained Energy

33. Mixed Bean Salad with Cherry Tomatoes

Ingredients:
- 1 (15 oz) can black beans, rinsed and drained
- 1 (15 oz) can kidney beans, rinsed and drained
- 1 (15 oz) can garbanzo beans (chickpeas), rinsed and drained
- 1 cup cherry tomatoes, halved
- 1/2 cup diced red onion
- 2 tablespoons chopped fresh parsley
- 2 tablespoons olive oil
- 2 tablespoons red wine vinegar
- 1 teaspoon Dijon mustard
- 1 clove garlic, minced
- Salt and black pepper to taste

PreparationTime: 15 minutes
Cook Time: 0 minutes
Total Time: 15 minutes
Serves: 4

Directions:
1. In a large bowl, combine the rinsed and drained black beans, kidney beans, and garbanzo beans.
2. Add the halved cherry tomatoes, diced red onion, and chopped fresh parsley.
3. In a small bowl, whisk together the olive oil, red wine vinegar, Dijon mustard, and minced garlic.
4. Pour the dressing over the bean and vegetable mixture and toss gently to coat.
5. Season with salt and black pepper to taste.
6. Serve chilled or at room temperature.

Storage Instructions:
The salad can be stored in an airtight container in the refrigerator for up to 4 days.

Variations and Tips:
- Use a variety of beans, such as lima beans or navy beans, for added texture and flavor.
- Add diced cucumber or bell pepper for extra crunch.
- Substitute fresh basil or cilantro for the parsley.
- Sprinkle with crumbled feta or shredded cheddar cheese.
- Serve the salad on a bed of mixed greens or with whole-grain crackers.

Nutrition Facts:

Calories: 260 - Total Fat: 8g - Saturated Fat: 1g - Cholesterol: 0mg - Sodium: 420mg
Total Carbohydrates: 36g - Dietary Fiber: 10g - Total Sugars: 4g - Protein: 12g

This mixed bean salad with cherry tomatoes is an excellent choice for managing type 2 diabetes. The combination of fiber-rich beans, low-glycemic cherry tomatoes, and healthy fats from the olive oil helps to regulate blood sugar levels and keep you feeling full and satisfied. The simple dressing provides flavor without added sugars. This salad can be enjoyed as a side dish or a light main course.

Lunch Recipes for Sustained Energy

34. Kale and Sweet Potato Salad

Ingredients:
- 2 medium sweet potatoes, peeled and cubed
- 1 tablespoon olive oil
- Salt and black pepper to taste
- 4 cups chopped kale, stems removed
- 1/2 cup diced red onion
- 1/4 cup toasted pumpkin seeds
- 2 tablespoons apple cider vinegar
- 1 tablespoon Dijon mustard
- 1 tablespoon honey
- 2 tablespoons olive oil

PreparationTime: 20 minutes
Cook Time: 25 minutes
Total Time: 45 minutes
Serves: 4

Directions:
1. Preheat the oven to 400°F (200°C).
2. Toss the cubed sweet potatoes with 1 tablespoon of olive oil and season with salt and black pepper.
3. Spread the sweet potatoes on a baking sheet and roast for 20-25 minutes, or until tender and lightly browned, stirring halfway through.
4. In a large salad bowl, combine the chopped kale, diced red onion, and toasted pumpkin seeds.
5. In a small bowl, whisk together the apple cider vinegar, Dijon mustard, honey, and 2 tablespoons of olive oil.
6. Add the roasted sweet potatoes to the kale mixture and drizzle the dressing over the top.
7. Toss the salad gently to coat the ingredients with the dressing.

Storage Instructions:
The roasted sweet potatoes can be stored in an airtight container in the refrigerator for up to 4 days. Assemble the salad just before serving for the best texture.

Variations and Tips:
- Use a mix of kale and spinach or arugula for a different flavor profile.
- Add diced avocado or crumbled feta cheese for extra creaminess.
- Substitute roasted chickpeas or almonds for the pumpkin seeds.
- Drizzle the salad with a tahini-based dressing or a balsamic vinaigrette.
- Serve the salad as a main course by adding grilled chicken or shrimp.

Nutrition Facts:
Calories: 240 - Total Fat: 12g - Saturated Fat: 2g - Cholesterol: 0mg - Sodium: 240mg
Total Carbohydrates: 29g - Dietary Fiber: 6g - Total Sugars: 9g - Protein: 6g

This kale and sweet potato salad is an excellent choice for managing type 2 diabetes. The sweet potatoes are a low-glycemic, nutrient-dense carbohydrate, while the kale provides a wealth of vitamins, minerals, and antioxidants. The pumpkin seeds add a crunchy texture and healthy fats, and the simple dressing is made with a small amount of honey to provide sweetness without spiking blood sugar levels.

Lunch Recipes for Sustained Energy

35. Chickpea and Avocado Sandwich

Ingredients:

- 1 (15 oz) can chickpeas, rinsed and drained
- 1/2 avocado, mashed
- 1 tablespoon lemon juice
- 1 tablespoon olive oil
- 1 teaspoon Dijon mustard
- 1/4 teaspoon garlic powder
- Salt and black pepper to taste
- 4 slices whole-grain bread
- 2 cups baby spinach leaves

PreparationTime: 10 minutes
Cook Time: 0 minutes
Total Time: 10 minutes
Serves: 2

Directions:

1. In a medium bowl, mash the chickpeas with a fork or potato masher.

2. Add the mashed avocado, lemon juice, olive oil, Dijon mustard, and garlic powder. Stir to combine.

3. Season the chickpea-avocado mixture with salt and black pepper to taste.

4. Divide the chickpea-avocado mixture evenly between 2 slices of whole-grain bread.

5. Top each sandwich with 1 cup of baby spinach leaves.

6. Place the remaining 2 slices of bread on top to create the sandwiches.

Storage Instructions:

The chickpea-avocado mixture can be stored in an airtight container in the refrigerator for up to 3 days. Assemble the sandwiches just before serving for the best texture.

Variations and Tips:

- Use a different type of bread, such as whole-wheat pita or a wrap, for variety.
- Add sliced tomatoes, cucumber, or red onion for extra crunch and flavor.
- Substitute roasted red pepper or sun-dried tomato hummus for the chickpea-avocado mixture.
- Serve the chickpea-avocado mixture on a bed of greens or with whole-grain crackers for a salad or snack option.
- For a heartier meal, add grilled chicken or turkey to the sandwich.

Nutrition Facts:

Calories: 350 - Total Fat: 16g - Saturated Fat: 2g - Cholesterol: 0mg
Sodium: 480mg - Total Carbohydrates: 42g - Dietary Fiber: 10g - Total Sugars: 4g - Protein: 12g

This chickpea and avocado sandwich is an excellent choice for managing type 2 diabetes. The chickpeas provide a good source of fiber and plant-based protein, while the avocado offers healthy fats and creaminess. The whole-grain bread and spinach leaves add additional fiber and nutrients. This sandwich can be enjoyed as a satisfying lunch or light dinner.

Lunch Recipes for Sustained Energy

36. Cabbage Slaw with Grilled Shrimp

Ingredients:

- 1 lb large shrimp, peeled and deveined
- 1 tablespoon olive oil
- 1 teaspoon paprika
- Salt and black pepper to taste
- 4 cups shredded green cabbage
- 1 cup shredded red cabbage
- 1/2 cup shredded carrots
- 1/4 cup chopped fresh cilantro
- 2 tablespoons apple cider vinegar
- 1 tablespoon olive oil
- 1 teaspoon Dijon mustard
- 1 teaspoon honey
- Salt and black pepper to taste

PreparationTime: 20 minutes
Cook Time: 10 minutes
Total Time: 30 minutes
Serves: 4

Directions:

1. Preheat grill or grill pan to medium-high heat.
2. In a medium bowl, toss the shrimp with 1 tablespoon of olive oil, paprika, salt, and black pepper.
3. Grill the shrimp for 2-3 minutes per side, or until cooked through. Set aside.
4. In a large bowl, combine the shredded green cabbage, red cabbage, carrots, and chopped fresh cilantro.
5. In a small bowl, whisk together the apple cider vinegar, 1 tablespoon of olive oil, Dijon mustard, and honey. Season with salt and black pepper to taste.
6. Pour the dressing over the cabbage slaw and toss to coat.
7. Divide the cabbage slaw among 4 plates and top each with grilled shrimp.

Storage Instructions:

The cabbage slaw can be stored in an airtight container in the refrigerator for up to 3 days. The grilled shrimp can be stored separately for up to 2 days.

Variations and Tips:

- Use a mix of green and red cabbage for a more colorful slaw.
- Add diced bell peppers, sliced radishes, or chopped green onions for extra crunch and flavor.
- Substitute grilled chicken or tofu for the shrimp for a different protein option.
- Serve the slaw and shrimp over a bed of mixed greens or with a side of quinoa or brown rice.
- Sprinkle the slaw with toasted almonds or sunflower seeds for added texture.

Nutrition Facts:

Calories: 220 - Total Fat: 9g - Saturated Fat: 1g - Cholesterol: 170mg - Sodium: 420mg
Total Carbohydrates: 14g - Dietary Fiber: 4g - Total Sugars: 7g - Protein: 22g

Lunch Recipes for Sustained Energy

37. Cauliflower Rice Bowl with Sautéed Vegetables

Ingredients:
- 1 head of cauliflower, cut into florets
- 1 tablespoon olive oil
- 1 red bell pepper, sliced
- 1 cup sliced mushrooms
- 1 cup broccoli florets
- 1 cup diced zucchini
- 2 cloves garlic, minced
- 1 tablespoon low-sodium soy sauce
- 1 tablespoon rice vinegar
- 1 teaspoon sesame oil
- Salt and black pepper to taste
- 2 tablespoons chopped fresh cilantro (optional)

PreparationTime: 20 minutes
Cook Time: 20 minutes
Total Time: 40 minutes
Serves: 4

Directions:
1. In a food processor, pulse the cauliflower florets until they resemble rice-sized grains. Set aside.
2. In a large skillet, heat the olive oil over medium-high heat. Add the sliced red bell pepper, mushrooms, broccoli florets, and diced zucchini. Sauté for 5-7 minutes, or until the vegetables are tender-crisp.
3. Add the minced garlic to the skillet and cook for an additional minute, stirring constantly.
4. Stir in the cauliflower rice, soy sauce, rice vinegar, and sesame oil. Cook for 5-7 minutes, or until the cauliflower rice is heated through and the flavors have combined.
5. Season the cauliflower rice bowl with salt and black pepper to taste.
6. Serve the cauliflower rice bowl warm, garnished with chopped fresh cilantro, if desired.

Storage Instructions:
The cauliflower rice bowl can be stored in an airtight container in the refrigerator for up to 4 days.

Variations and Tips:
- Use a mix of vegetables, such as carrots, snow peas, or spinach, for added variety.
- Add cooked chicken, shrimp, or tofu for extra protein.
- Substitute tamari or coconut aminos for the soy sauce for a gluten-free option.
- Top the bowl with a fried or poached egg for a more substantial meal.
- Serve the cauliflower rice bowl with a side of roasted nuts or seeds for added crunch and healthy fats.

Nutrition Facts:

Calories: 120 - Total Fat: 5g - Saturated Fat: 1g - Cholesterol: 0mg - Sodium: 260mg
Total Carbohydrates: 14g - Dietary Fiber: 5g - Total Sugars: 5g - Protein: 5g

Lunch Recipes for Sustained Energy

38. Tomato Basil Soup with a Side Salad

Ingredients:

Tomato Basil Soup:
- 1 tablespoon olive oil
- 1 onion, diced
- 3 cloves garlic, minced
- 1 (28 oz) can diced tomatoes
- 2 cups low-sodium vegetable broth
- 1/4 cup fresh basil, chopped
- 1 teaspoon dried oregano
- Salt and black pepper to taste

Side Salad:
- 4 cups mixed greens
- 1 cup cherry tomatoes, halved
- 1/4 cup sliced cucumber
- 2 tablespoons balsamic vinegar
- 1 tablespoon olive oil
- Salt and black pepper to taste

PreparationTime: 20 minutes
Cook Time: 30 minutes
Total Time: 50 minutes
Serves: 4

Directions:

Tomato Basil Soup:
1. In a large saucepan, heat the olive oil over medium heat. Add the diced onion and sauté for 5 minutes, or until translucent.
2. Add the minced garlic and sauté for an additional minute, until fragrant.
3. Stir in the diced tomatoes, vegetable broth, chopped fresh basil, and dried oregano. Season with salt and black pepper to taste.
4. Bring the soup to a simmer and cook for 20-25 minutes, or until the flavors have melded.
5. Using an immersion blender or a regular blender, puree the soup until smooth.

Side Salad:
1. In a large salad bowl, combine the mixed greens, halved cherry tomatoes, and sliced cucumber.
2. In a small bowl, whisk together the balsamic vinegar and olive oil. Season with salt and black pepper to taste.
3. Drizzle the dressing over the salad and toss gently to coat.

Serve the tomato basil soup warm, with the side salad on the side.

Storage Instructions:
The tomato basil soup can be stored in an airtight container in the refrigerator for up to 4 days. The side salad can be prepared and stored separately for up to 2 days.

Lunch Recipes for Sustained Energy

39. Spinach and Feta Stuffed Peppers

Ingredients:
- 4 medium bell peppers, halved lengthwise and seeded
- 1 tablespoon olive oil
- 1 onion, diced
- 2 cloves garlic, minced
- 5 oz baby spinach, chopped
- 1 cup crumbled feta cheese
- 1/4 cup grated Parmesan cheese
- 1 teaspoon dried oregano
- Salt and black pepper to taste

PreparationTime: 20 minutes
Cook Time: 30 minutes
Total Time: 50 minutes
Serves: 4

Directions:
1. Preheat the oven to 375°F (190°C).
2. Place the bell pepper halves, cut-side up, in a baking dish. Set aside.
3. In a skillet, heat the olive oil over medium heat. Add the diced onion and sauté for 5 minutes, or until translucent.
4. Add the minced garlic and chopped spinach to the skillet. Cook for 2-3 minutes, or until the spinach is wilted.
5. Remove the skillet from heat and stir in the crumbled feta cheese, grated Parmesan cheese, and dried oregano. Season with salt and black pepper to taste.
6. Spoon the spinach and feta mixture evenly into the bell pepper halves.
7. Bake the stuffed peppers for 25-30 minutes, or until the peppers are tender and the filling is hot and bubbly.

Storage Instructions:
The stuffed peppers can be stored in an airtight container in the refrigerator for up to 3 days.

Variations and Tips:
- Use a variety of bell peppers, such as red, yellow, or orange, for a more colorful dish.
- Add diced tomatoes or sun-dried tomatoes to the filling for extra flavor.
- Substitute goat cheese or shredded mozzarella for the feta cheese.
- Sprinkle the tops of the stuffed peppers with breadcrumbs or crushed nuts for a crunchy topping.
- Serve the stuffed peppers with a side salad or a small portion of whole-grain rice or quinoa.

Nutrition Facts:
Calories: 180 - Total Fat: 10g - Saturated Fat: 5g - Cholesterol: 25mg - Sodium: 420mg
Total Carbohydrates: 14g - Dietary Fiber: 4g - Total Sugars: 6g - Protein: 12g

These spinach and feta stuffed peppers are an excellent choice for managing type 2 diabetes. The bell peppers are a low-glycemic vegetable, while the spinach and feta cheese provide a nutrient-dense and protein-rich filling. The small amount of Parmesan cheese adds flavor without significantly increasing the saturated fat or sodium content. This dish is a satisfying and balanced meal option.

Lunch Recipes for Sustained Energy

40. Chicken and Broccoli Stir-Fry

Ingredients:

- 1 lb boneless, skinless chicken breasts, cut into 1-inch pieces
- 2 tablespoons low-sodium soy sauce
- 1 tablespoon rice vinegar
- 1 teaspoon sesame oil
- 1 tablespoon olive oil
- 3 cloves garlic, minced
- 1 inch piece fresh ginger, peeled and grated
- 4 cups broccoli florets
- 1/2 cup low-sodium chicken broth
- 1 tablespoon cornstarch
- Salt and black pepper to taste
- 2 cups cooked brown rice, for serving

PreparationTime: 15 minutes
Cook Time: 20 minutes
Total Time: 35 minutes
Serves: 4

Directions:

1. In a medium bowl, combine the cubed chicken, low-sodium soy sauce, rice vinegar, and sesame oil. Toss to coat the chicken and set aside.
2. In a large skillet or wok, heat the olive oil over medium-high heat. Add the minced garlic and grated ginger and cook for 1 minute, stirring constantly, until fragrant.
3. Add the broccoli florets to the skillet and stir-fry for 3-4 minutes, or until the broccoli is starting to soften.
4. In a small bowl, whisk together the low-sodium chicken broth and cornstarch.
5. Add the marinated chicken to the skillet and cook for 5-7 minutes, or until the chicken is cooked through.
6. Pour the chicken broth and cornstarch mixture into the skillet and stir to combine. Cook for an additional 2-3 minutes, or until the sauce has thickened.
7. Season the stir-fry with salt and black pepper to taste.
8. Serve the chicken and broccoli stir-fry over the cooked brown rice.

Storage Instructions:

The stir-fry can be stored in an airtight container in the refrigerator for up to 4 days.

Variations and Tips:

- Add sliced mushrooms, bell peppers, or snow peas for extra vegetables.
- Use low-sodium tamari or coconut aminos instead of soy sauce for a gluten-free option.
- Substitute tofu or shrimp for the chicken for a different protein source.
- Serve the stir-fry with cauliflower rice or zucchini noodles for a lower-carb alternative.
- Sprinkle the dish with chopped green onions, toasted sesame seeds, or crushed red pepper flakes for added flavor.

Nutrition Facts:

Calories: 300 - Total Fat: 9g - Saturated Fat: 1.5g - Cholesterol: 70mg - Sodium: 420mg
Total Carbohydrates: 27g - Dietary Fiber: 5g - Total Sugars: 3g - Protein: 30g

Lunch Recipes for Sustained Energy

41. Baked Salmon with Quinoa and Steamed Broccoli

Ingredients:
- 4 (6 oz) salmon fillets
- 1 tablespoon olive oil
- 1 teaspoon lemon zest
- 1 tablespoon lemon juice
- Salt and black pepper to taste
- 1 cup uncooked quinoa, rinsed
- 2 cups low-sodium chicken or vegetable broth
- 4 cups broccoli florets
- 1 tablespoon unsalted butter (optional)

PreparationTime: 15 minutes
Cook Time: 30 minutes
Total Time: 45 minutes
Serves: 4

Directions:
1. Preheat the oven to 400°F (200°C).
2. Place the salmon fillets on a baking sheet lined with parchment paper. Drizzle with the olive oil and sprinkle with the lemon zest, lemon juice, salt, and black pepper.
3. Bake the salmon for 15-20 minutes, or until it flakes easily with a fork.
4. While the salmon is baking, cook the quinoa. In a medium saucepan, combine the rinsed quinoa and broth. Bring to a boil, then reduce heat to low, cover, and simmer for 15-20 minutes, or until the quinoa is tender and the liquid is absorbed.
5. In a steamer basket or saucepan with a small amount of water, steam the broccoli florets for 5-7 minutes, or until tender-crisp.
6. Serve the baked salmon fillets over the cooked quinoa, with the steamed broccoli on the side. If desired, top the broccoli with a small amount of unsalted butter.

Storage Instructions: The baked salmon, cooked quinoa, and steamed broccoli can be stored separately in airtight containers in the refrigerator for up to 3 days.

Variations and Tips:
- Use a different type of fish, such as halibut or cod, if desired.
- Roast the broccoli instead of steaming it for a different texture.
- Add diced avocado or a drizzle of pesto to the quinoa for extra flavor.
- Serve the meal with a side salad or a small portion of roasted sweet potatoes.
- Sprinkle the salmon or broccoli with chopped fresh herbs, such as dill or parsley, before serving.

Nutrition Facts:
Calories: 420 - Total Fat: 18g - Saturated Fat: 4g - Cholesterol: 90mg - Sodium: 240mg
Total Carbohydrates: 32g - Dietary Fiber: 6g - Total Sugars: 2g - Protein: 35g

This baked salmon with quinoa and steamed broccoli is an excellent choice for managing type 2 diabetes. Salmon is a rich source of omega-3 fatty acids, which can help improve insulin sensitivity and reduce inflammation. Quinoa is a high-fiber, low-glycemic grain that provides complex carbohydrates, and the steamed broccoli is a nutrient-dense vegetable. This well-balanced meal is a great option for maintaining healthy blood sugar levels.

Dinner Recipes for Balanced Nutrition

42. Chicken Stir-Fry with Snap Peas and Brown Rice

Ingredients:

- 1 lb boneless, skinless chicken breasts, cut into 1-inch pieces
- 2 tablespoons low-sodium soy sauce
- 1 tablespoon rice vinegar
- 1 teaspoon sesame oil
- 1 tablespoon olive oil
- 3 cloves garlic, minced
- 1 inch piece fresh ginger, peeled and grated
- 2 cups snap peas, trimmed
- 1 red bell pepper, sliced
- 1/2 cup low-sodium chicken broth
- 1 tablespoon cornstarch
- Salt and black pepper to taste
- 2 cups cooked brown rice, for serving

PreparationTime: 20 minutes
Cook Time: 20 minutes
Total Time: 40 minutes
Serves: 4

Directions:

1. In a medium bowl, combine the cubed chicken, low-sodium soy sauce, rice vinegar, and sesame oil. Toss to coat the chicken and set aside.
2. In a large skillet or wok, heat the olive oil over medium-high heat. Add the minced garlic and grated ginger and cook for 1 minute, stirring constantly, until fragrant.
3. Add the snap peas and sliced red bell pepper to the skillet and stir-fry for 3-4 minutes, or until the vegetables are starting to soften.
4. Add the marinated chicken to the skillet and cook for 5-7 minutes, or until the chicken is cooked through.
5. In a small bowl, whisk together the low-sodium chicken broth and cornstarch.
6. Pour the chicken broth and cornstarch mixture into the skillet and stir to combine. Cook for an additional 2-3 minutes, or until the sauce has thickened.
7. Season the stir-fry with salt and black pepper to taste.
8. Serve the chicken and vegetable stir-fry over the cooked brown rice.

Storage Instructions:

The stir-fry can be stored in an airtight container in the refrigerator for up to 4 days.

Variations and Tips:
- Add sliced mushrooms, water chestnuts, or baby corn for extra vegetables.
- Use low-sodium tamari or coconut aminos instead of soy sauce for a gluten-free option.
- Substitute tofu or shrimp for the chicken for a different protein source.
- Serve the stir-fry with cauliflower rice or zucchini noodles for a lower-carb alternative.
- Sprinkle the dish with chopped green onions, toasted sesame seeds, or crushed red pepper flakes for added flavor.

Nutrition Facts:

Calories: 330 - Total Fat: 10g - Saturated Fat: 2g - Cholesterol: 70mg - Sodium: 420mg
Total Carbohydrates: 32g - Dietary Fiber: 5g - Total Sugars: 4g - Protein: 30g

Dinner Recipes for Balanced Nutrition

43. Baked Cod with Lemon and Dill

Ingredients:
- 4 (6 oz) cod fillets
- 2 tablespoons olive oil
- 2 tablespoons lemon juice
- 2 tablespoons chopped fresh dill
- 1 teaspoon grated lemon zest
- Salt and black pepper to taste
- 1 lemon, cut into wedges for serving

PreparationTime: 10 minutes
Cook Time: 20 minutes
Total Time: 30 minutes
Serves: 4

Directions:

1. Preheat the oven to 400°F (200°C).

2. Place the cod fillets in a baking dish or on a parchment-lined baking sheet.

3. In a small bowl, whisk together the olive oil, lemon juice, chopped fresh dill, and lemon zest.

4. Drizzle the lemon-dill mixture over the cod fillets and use a brush or your fingers to evenly coat the fish.

5. Season the cod with salt and black pepper to taste.

6. Bake the cod for 15-20 minutes, or until it flakes easily with a fork.

7. Serve the baked cod warm, with lemon wedges on the side.

Storage Instructions:
The baked cod can be stored in an airtight container in the refrigerator for up to 3 days.

Variations and Tips:
- Use a different type of white fish, such as halibut or tilapia, if desired.
- Add sliced cherry tomatoes or diced cucumber to the baking dish for extra flavor and nutrients.
- Sprinkle the cod with a small amount of grated Parmesan cheese or breadcrumbs before baking for a crispy topping.
- Serve the baked cod over a bed of steamed vegetables, such as broccoli or asparagus.
- Squeeze additional lemon juice over the cod just before serving for a bright, fresh flavor.

Nutrition Facts:

Calories: 220 - Total Fat: 9g - Saturated Fat: 1.5g - Cholesterol: 70mg
Sodium: 150mg - Total Carbohydrates: 1g - Dietary Fiber: 0g - Total Sugars: 0g - Protein: 30g

This baked cod with lemon and dill is an excellent choice for managing type 2 diabetes. Cod is a lean, high-protein fish that is low in carbohydrates and calories. The lemon and dill provide fresh, bright flavors without the need for added sugars or unhealthy fats. This simple, yet delicious, dish is a great option for a healthy, diabetes-friendly meal.

Dinner Recipes for Balanced Nutrition

44. Turkey Meatballs with Zucchini Noodles

Ingredients:
Meatballs:
- 1 lb ground turkey
- 1/4 cup whole-wheat breadcrumbs
- 1 egg, beaten
- 2 tablespoons grated Parmesan cheese
- 2 cloves garlic, minced
- 1 teaspoon dried oregano
- Salt and black pepper to taste

Zucchini Noodles:
- 3 medium zucchini, spiralized or julienned
- 1 tablespoon olive oil
- 2 cloves garlic, minced
- 1 (24 oz) jar low-sodium marinara sauce
- 2 tablespoons chopped fresh basil

PreparationTime: 20 minutes
Cook Time: 25 minutes
Total Time: 45 minutes
Serves: 4

Directions:
Meatballs:
1. Preheat the oven to 400°F (200°C).
2. In a medium bowl, combine the ground turkey, whole-wheat breadcrumbs, beaten egg, grated Parmesan cheese, minced garlic, and dried oregano. Season with salt and black pepper.
3. Roll the mixture into 1-inch meatballs and place them on a baking sheet lined with parchment paper. Bake the meatballs for 20-25 minutes, or until cooked through.

Zucchini Noodles:
1. In a large skillet, heat the olive oil over medium heat. Add the minced garlic and sauté for 1 minute, until fragrant.
2. Add the spiralized or julienned zucchini noodles to the skillet and sauté for 3-5 minutes, or until the noodles are tender-crisp.
3. Pour the low-sodium marinara sauce over the zucchini noodles and heat through.
4. Serve the turkey meatballs over the zucchini noodles, garnished with chopped fresh basil.

Storage Instructions:
The cooked meatballs and zucchini noodles can be stored separately in airtight containers in the refrigerator for up to 3 days.

Variations and Tips:
- Use ground chicken or lean ground beef instead of turkey for a different protein option.
- Add grated carrots or diced bell peppers to the meatball mixture for extra vegetables.
- Substitute pesto or a low-sugar tomato sauce for the marinara sauce.
- Serve the meatballs and zucchini noodles with a side salad or roasted vegetables.
- Top the dish with grated Parmesan cheese or a sprinkle of crushed red pepper flakes.

Dinner Recipes for Balanced Nutrition

45. Beef and Vegetable Kebabs

Ingredients:
- 1 lb beef sirloin, cut into 1-inch cubes
- 1 red bell pepper, cut into 1-inch pieces
- 1 yellow bell pepper, cut into 1-inch pieces
- 1 zucchini, cut into 1-inch pieces
- 1 red onion, cut into 1-inch pieces
- 2 tablespoons olive oil
- 2 tablespoons balsamic vinegar
- 1 teaspoon dried oregano
- 1/2 teaspoon garlic powder
- Salt and black pepper to taste

PreparationTime: 20 minutes
Cook Time: 15 minutes
Total Time: 35 minutes
Serves: 4

Directions:
1. Preheat grill or grill pan to medium-high heat.

2. In a large bowl, combine the beef, bell peppers, zucchini, and onion. Drizzle with olive oil and balsamic vinegar, then sprinkle with oregano, garlic powder, salt, and black pepper. Toss to coat the ingredients evenly.

3. Thread the beef and vegetables onto skewers, alternating the ingredients.

4. Grill the kebabs for 12-15 minutes, turning occasionally, until the beef is cooked through and the vegetables are tender.

5. Serve hot.

Storage Instructions:
- Leftovers can be stored in an airtight container in the refrigerator for up to 3 days.

Variations and Tips:
- Use different types of vegetables, such as mushrooms, cherry tomatoes, or eggplant.

- Marinate the beef in the balsamic vinegar mixture for 30 minutes to 1 hour before assembling the kebabs for more flavor.

- Soak wooden skewers in water for 30 minutes before using to prevent them from burning.

- Serve the kebabs with rice, quinoa, or a fresh salad for a complete meal.

Nutrition Facts:
Calories: 250 | Total Fat: 12g | Saturated Fat: 3g | Cholesterol: 60mg | Sodium: 150mg | Total Carbohydrates: 12g | Dietary Fiber: 3g | Total Sugars: 6g | Protein: 25g

Dinner Recipes for Balanced Nutrition

46. Stuffed Bell Peppers with Ground Turkey and Quinoa

Ingredients:
- 4 medium bell peppers (any color)
- 1 lb ground turkey
- 1 cup cooked quinoa
- 1 small onion, diced
- 2 cloves garlic, minced
- 1 (14.5 oz) can diced tomatoes
- 1 tsp dried oregano
- 1/2 tsp ground cumin
- 1/4 tsp cayenne pepper (optional)
- Salt and black pepper to taste
- 1/2 cup shredded low-fat cheddar cheese (optional)

PreparationTime: 20 minutes
Cook Time: 40 minutes
Total Time: 1 hour
Serves: 4

Directions:
1. Preheat oven to 375°F.
2. Cut the tops off the bell peppers and remove the seeds and membranes. Place the peppers in a baking dish and set aside.
3. In a large skillet, cook the ground turkey over medium heat until browned, 5-7 minutes, making sure to crumble the meat as it cooks.
4. Add the onion and garlic to the skillet and cook for 2-3 minutes, until the onion is translucent.
5. Stir in the cooked quinoa, diced tomatoes, oregano, cumin, cayenne (if using), salt, and black pepper. Cook for 5 minutes, stirring occasionally.
6. Spoon the turkey-quinoa mixture into the hollowed-out bell peppers. Top with shredded cheese, if desired.
7. Bake for 30-35 minutes, or until the peppers are tender and the filling is hot.
8. Serve hot.

Storage Instructions:
- Leftovers can be stored in an airtight container in the refrigerator for up to 3 days.

Variations and Tips:
- Use different types of ground meat, such as chicken or lean beef, if desired.
- Add diced vegetables, such as zucchini or spinach, to the filling for extra nutrition.
- Serve the stuffed peppers with a side salad or roasted vegetables for a complete meal.

Nutrition Facts:
Calories: 300 | Total Fat: 12g | Saturated Fat: 3g | Cholesterol: 75mg | Sodium: 450mg | Total Carbohydrates: 22g | Dietary Fiber: 5g | Total Sugars: 7g | Protein: 28g

This recipe is a great option for managing type 2 diabetes, as it is high in protein, fiber, and complex carbohydrates, while being low in saturated fat and sodium. The bell peppers provide a good source of vitamins and minerals, and the quinoa adds a boost of fiber and nutrients.

Dinner Recipes for Balanced Nutrition

47. Grilled Chicken with Mango Salsa

Ingredients:

Mango Salsa:
- 1 ripe mango, diced
- 1/2 red onion, finely chopped
- 1 jalapeño, seeded and finely chopped
- 1/4 cup chopped fresh cilantro
- 2 tablespoons lime juice
- 1/4 teaspoon salt

Grilled Chicken:
- 4 boneless, skinless chicken breasts
- 1 tablespoon olive oil
- 1 teaspoon chili powder
- 1/2 teaspoon garlic powder
- 1/4 teaspoon salt
- 1/4 teaspoon black pepper

PreparationTime: 20 minutes
Cook Time: 15 minutes
Total Time: 35 minutes
Serves: 4

Directions:

1. Make the mango salsa: In a medium bowl, combine the diced mango, red onion, jalapeño, cilantro, lime juice, and 1/4 teaspoon of salt. Stir to mix well and set aside.
2. Prepare the chicken: Preheat grill or grill pan to medium-high heat.
3. Brush the chicken breasts with olive oil and season with chili powder, garlic powder, salt, and black pepper.
4. Grill the chicken for 6-8 minutes per side, or until cooked through and no longer pink in the center.
5. Serve the grilled chicken topped with the mango salsa.

Storage Instructions:

- Leftover chicken and salsa can be stored separately in airtight containers in the refrigerator for up to 3 days.

Variations and Tips:

- Use different types of fruit, such as pineapple or peach, in the salsa.
- Add diced avocado to the salsa for extra creaminess.
- Serve the chicken and salsa over a bed of mixed greens or with a side of roasted vegetables.

Nutrition Facts:

Calories: 250 | Total Fat: 8g | Saturated Fat: 2g | Cholesterol: 90mg | Sodium: 400mg | Total Carbohydrates: 15g | Dietary Fiber: 3g | Total Sugars: 12g | Protein: 30g

This recipe is a great option for managing type 2 diabetes, as it is high in protein, low in carbohydrates, and features a fresh, flavorful salsa made with nutrient-dense ingredients like mango and cilantro. The grilled chicken provides a lean protein source, while the mango salsa adds a burst of sweetness and acidity to balance the dish.

Dinner Recipes for Balanced Nutrition

48. Pork Tenderloin with Roasted Brussels Sprouts

Ingredients:

Pork Tenderloin:
- 1 lb pork tenderloin
- 1 tablespoon olive oil
- 1 teaspoon garlic powder
- 1 teaspoon dried thyme
- 1/2 teaspoon salt
- 1/4 teaspoon black pepper

Roasted Brussels Sprouts:
- 1 lb Brussels sprouts, trimmed and halved
- 2 tablespoons olive oil
- 1/2 teaspoon salt
- 1/4 teaspoon black pepper

PreparationTime: 15 minutes
Cook Time: 30 minutes
Total Time: 45 minutes
Serves: 4

Directions:

1. Preheat oven to 400°F.
2. Prepare the pork tenderloin: Rub the pork tenderloin with olive oil, garlic powder, dried thyme, salt, and black pepper.
3. Place the pork tenderloin on a baking sheet and roast for 20-25 minutes, or until the internal temperature reaches 145°F.
4. While the pork is roasting, prepare the Brussels sprouts: Toss the Brussels sprouts with olive oil, salt, and black pepper on a separate baking sheet.
5. Roast the Brussels sprouts for 15-20 minutes, or until they are tender and lightly browned.
6. Remove the pork tenderloin and Brussels sprouts from the oven and let the pork rest for 5 minutes before slicing.
7. Serve the sliced pork tenderloin with the roasted Brussels sprouts.

Storage Instructions:

- Leftover pork and Brussels sprouts can be stored separately in airtight containers in the refrigerator for up to 3 days.

Variations and Tips:

- Roast the Brussels sprouts with other vegetables, such as carrots, parsnips, or sweet potatoes, for added flavor and nutrition.
- Drizzle the roasted Brussels sprouts with a balsamic glaze or lemon juice for extra flavor.
- Serve the pork and Brussels sprouts with a side of quinoa or brown rice for a more complete meal.

Nutrition Facts:

Calories: 300 | Total Fat: 12g | Saturated Fat: 2g | Cholesterol: 90mg | Sodium: 550mg | Total Carbohydrates: 15g | Dietary Fiber: 5g | Total Sugars: 4g | Protein: 35g

Dinner Recipes for Balanced Nutrition

49. Shrimp Scampi with Whole Wheat Pasta

Ingredients:
- 8 oz whole wheat pasta (such as spaghetti or linguine)
- 1 lb shrimp, peeled and deveined
- 2 tablespoons olive oil
- 3 cloves garlic, minced
- 1/4 cup dry white wine or low-sodium chicken broth
- 2 tablespoons lemon juice
- 2 tablespoons chopped fresh parsley
- 1/4 teaspoon red pepper flakes (optional)
- Salt and black pepper to taste

Preparation Time: 15 minutes
Cook Time: 20 minutes
Total Time: 35 minutes
Serves: 4

Directions:
1. Bring a large pot of salted water to a boil. Cook the whole wheat pasta according to package instructions, until al dente. Drain and set aside.
2. In a large skillet, heat the olive oil over medium heat. Add the garlic and cook for 1 minute, until fragrant.
3. Add the shrimp to the skillet and cook for 2-3 minutes per side, or until the shrimp are pink and opaque.
4. Deglaze the pan with the white wine or chicken broth, scraping up any browned bits from the bottom of the pan.
5. Stir in the lemon juice, parsley, and red pepper flakes (if using). Season with salt and black pepper to taste.
6. Add the cooked whole wheat pasta to the skillet and toss to combine.
7. Serve the shrimp scampi with whole wheat pasta immediately.

Storage Instructions:
- Leftover shrimp scampi with pasta can be stored in an airtight container in the refrigerator for up to 3 days.

Variations and Tips:
- Use a combination of shrimp and scallops for added seafood flavor.
- Add diced tomatoes or spinach to the skillet for extra nutrition.
- Serve the shrimp scampi over zucchini noodles or cauliflower rice for a lower-carb option.

Nutrition Facts:
Calories: 350 | Total Fat: 10g | Saturated Fat: 2g | Cholesterol: 200mg | Sodium: 450mg | Total Carbohydrates: 35g | Dietary Fiber: 6g | Total Sugars: 3g | Protein: 30g

This recipe is a great option for managing type 2 diabetes, as it features whole wheat pasta, which is a good source of complex carbohydrates, fiber, and nutrients. The shrimp provide a lean protein source, while the garlic, lemon, and parsley add flavor without the need for excessive salt or butter.

Dinner Recipes for Balanced Nutrition

50. Lentil and Spinach Stew

Ingredients:
- 1 tablespoon olive oil
- 1 onion, diced
- 3 cloves garlic, minced
- 1 cup brown or green lentils, rinsed
- 4 cups low-sodium vegetable or chicken broth
- 1 (14.5 oz) can diced tomatoes
- 1 teaspoon ground cumin
- 1/2 teaspoon dried thyme
- 1/4 teaspoon cayenne pepper (optional)
- Salt and black pepper to taste
- 4 cups fresh spinach, chopped

PreparationTime: 15 minutes
Cook Time: 30 minutes
Total Time: 45 minutes
Serves: 4

Directions:
1. In a large pot or Dutch oven, heat the olive oil over medium heat. Add the onion and sauté for 5 minutes, until translucent.
2. Add the garlic and sauté for 1 minute, until fragrant.
3. Stir in the lentils, broth, diced tomatoes, cumin, thyme, and cayenne pepper (if using). Season with salt and black pepper to taste.
4. Bring the mixture to a boil, then reduce the heat and simmer for 20-25 minutes, or until the lentils are tender.
5. Stir in the chopped spinach and cook for an additional 5 minutes, or until the spinach is wilted.
6. Serve the lentil and spinach stew hot.

Storage Instructions:
- Leftover stew can be stored in an airtight container in the refrigerator for up to 4 days.

Variations and Tips:
- Add diced carrots, celery, or other vegetables to the stew for extra nutrition.
- Use a combination of lentils, such as red and green, for a more varied texture.
- Serve the stew with a side of whole grain bread or crackers for a more filling meal.

Nutrition Facts:
Calories: 250 | Total Fat: 5g | Saturated Fat: 1g | Cholesterol: 0mg | Sodium: 450mg | Total Carbohydrates: 35g | Dietary Fiber: 12g | Total Sugars: 6g | Protein: 15g

This lentil and spinach stew is an excellent choice for managing type 2 diabetes. Lentils are a great source of fiber, protein, and complex carbohydrates, while spinach provides a nutrient-dense vegetable. The stew is low in calories, fat, and sodium, making it a healthy and satisfying meal option.

Dinner Recipes for Balanced Nutrition

51. Baked Tilapia with Green Beans

Ingredients:
- 4 (6 oz) tilapia fillets
- 1 tablespoon olive oil
- 1 teaspoon garlic powder
- 1 teaspoon paprika
- 1/2 teaspoon salt
- 1/4 teaspoon black pepper
- 1 lb green beans, trimmed
- 1 tablespoon lemon juice
- 2 tablespoons chopped fresh parsley (optional)

PreparationTime: 10 minutes
Cook Time: 20 minutes
Total Time: 30 minutes
Serves: 4

Directions:
1. Preheat oven to 400°F. Line a baking sheet with parchment paper or foil.
2. Place the tilapia fillets on the prepared baking sheet. Drizzle with olive oil and sprinkle with garlic powder, paprika, salt, and black pepper.
3. Arrange the green beans around the tilapia fillets.
4. Bake for 15-20 minutes, or until the fish is cooked through and flakes easily with a fork, and the green beans are tender.
5. Remove the baked tilapia and green beans from the oven. Drizzle the lemon juice over the fish and vegetables.
6. Garnish with chopped fresh parsley, if desired.
7. Serve immediately.

Storage Instructions:
- Leftover baked tilapia and green beans can be stored in an airtight container in the refrigerator for up to 3 days.

Variations and Tips:
- Use other types of white fish, such as cod or halibut, in place of tilapia.
- Roast the green beans with other vegetables, such as cherry tomatoes or sliced zucchini.
- Serve the baked tilapia and green beans with a side of quinoa or brown rice for a more complete meal.

Nutrition Facts:
Calories: 200 | Total Fat: 6g | Saturated Fat: 1g | Cholesterol: 70mg | Sodium: 400mg | Total Carbohydrates: 10g | Dietary Fiber: 4g | Total Sugars: 3g | Protein: 28g

This baked tilapia with green beans recipe is an excellent choice for managing type 2 diabetes. Tilapia is a lean, low-calorie protein source, while the green beans provide fiber, vitamins, and minerals. The simple seasoning and baking method keep the dish light and healthy, making it a great option for a balanced meal.

52. Chicken and Mushroom Risotto

Ingredients:
- 4 cups low-sodium chicken broth
- 1 tablespoon olive oil
- 1 lb boneless, skinless chicken breasts, cut into 1-inch pieces
- 8 oz sliced mushrooms
- 1 onion, diced
- 2 cloves garlic, minced
- 1 cup Arborio rice
- 1/2 cup dry white wine (or additional chicken broth)
- 1/4 cup grated Parmesan cheese
- 2 tablespoons chopped fresh parsley
- Salt and black pepper to taste

PreparationTime: 15 minutes
Cook Time: 30 minutes
Total Time: 45 minutes
Serves: 4

Directions:
1. In a saucepan, bring the chicken broth to a simmer and keep it warm over low heat.
2. In a large skillet, heat the olive oil over medium-high heat. Add the chicken and cook for 3-4 minutes, until lightly browned. Remove the chicken from the skillet and set aside.
3. Add the mushrooms, onion, and garlic to the skillet. Cook for 5-7 minutes, stirring occasionally, until the vegetables are softened.
4. Add the Arborio rice to the skillet and stir to coat the grains with the oil. Cook for 2-3 minutes, until the rice is slightly toasted.
5. Pour in the white wine (or additional chicken broth) and stir, scraping up any browned bits from the bottom of the skillet. Cook for 2-3 minutes, until the liquid is mostly absorbed.
6. Ladle in 1/2 cup of the warm chicken broth and stir constantly until the liquid is absorbed. Continue this process, adding 1/2 cup of broth at a time, until the rice is tender and creamy, about 20-25 minutes total.
7. Stir the cooked chicken back into the risotto, along with the Parmesan cheese and parsley. Season with salt and black pepper to taste.
8. Serve the chicken and mushroom risotto immediately.

Storage Instructions: - Leftover risotto can be stored in an airtight container in the refrigerator for up to 3 days.

Variations and Tips:
- Use a combination of mushrooms, such as cremini and shiitake, for added flavor.
- Stir in a handful of baby spinach or kale at the end for extra nutrition.
- Serve the risotto with a side salad for a complete meal.

Nutrition Facts:
Calories: 350 | Total Fat: 10g | Saturated Fat: 3g | Cholesterol: 70mg | Sodium: 450mg | Total Carbohydrates: 35g | Dietary Fiber: 3g | Total Sugars: 3g | Protein: 30g

Dinner Recipes for Balanced Nutrition

53. Spaghetti Squash with Marinara Sauce and Turkey Meatballs

Ingredients:
Spaghetti Squash:
- 1 medium spaghetti squash, halved lengthwise and seeded
- 1 tablespoon olive oil
- Salt and black pepper to taste

Turkey Meatballs:
- 1 lb ground turkey
- 1/4 cup whole wheat breadcrumbs
- 1 egg, lightly beaten
- 2 tablespoons grated Parmesan cheese
- 2 cloves garlic, minced
- 1 teaspoon dried oregano
- 1/4 teaspoon salt
- 1/4 teaspoon black pepper

Marinara Sauce:
- 1 (28 oz) can crushed tomatoes
- 2 cloves garlic, minced
- 1 teaspoon dried basil
- 1/4 teaspoon red pepper flakes (optional)
- Salt and black pepper to taste

PreparationTime: 20 minutes
Cook Time: 45 minutes
Total Time: 1 hour 5 minutes
Serves: 4

Directions:
1. Preheat oven to 400°F.
2. Prepare the spaghetti squash: Place the halved squash cut-side up on a baking sheet. Drizzle with olive oil and season with salt and black pepper. Roast for 35-45 minutes, or until the squash is tender and easily shreds with a fork.
3. Make the turkey meatballs: In a large bowl, combine the ground turkey, breadcrumbs, egg, Parmesan, garlic, oregano, salt, and black pepper. Mix well and form into 12 equal-sized meatballs.
4. Place the meatballs on a separate baking sheet and bake for 20-25 minutes, or until cooked through.
5. Prepare the marinara sauce: In a saucepan, combine the crushed tomatoes, garlic, basil, and red pepper flakes (if using). Season with salt and black pepper to taste. Simmer for 10 minutes.
6. Use a fork to shred the roasted spaghetti squash into strands.
7. Serve the spaghetti squash topped with the marinara sauce and turkey meatballs.

Storage Instructions:
- Leftover spaghetti squash, meatballs, and sauce can be stored separately in airtight containers in the refrigerator for up to 3 days.

Dinner Recipes for Balanced Nutrition

54. Grilled Eggplant with Tomato and Feta

Ingredients:
- 1 medium eggplant, sliced into 1/2-inch thick rounds
- 2 tablespoons olive oil, plus more for brushing
- 1 pint cherry tomatoes, halved
- 1/2 cup crumbled feta cheese
- 2 tablespoons chopped fresh basil
- 1 tablespoon balsamic vinegar
- 1/4 teaspoon salt
- 1/4 teaspoon black pepper

PreparationTime: 15 minutes
Cook Time: 20 minutes
Total Time: 35 minutes
Serves: 4

Directions:
1. Preheat grill or grill pan to medium-high heat.
2. Brush the eggplant slices with olive oil on both sides and season with salt and black pepper.
3. Grill the eggplant slices for 3-4 minutes per side, or until tender and lightly charred.
4. In a medium bowl, combine the halved cherry tomatoes, feta cheese, basil, balsamic vinegar, 2 tablespoons of olive oil, salt, and black pepper. Toss to mix well.
5. Arrange the grilled eggplant slices on a serving platter or plate. Top with the tomato-feta mixture.
6. Serve immediately.

Storage Instructions:
- Leftover grilled eggplant and tomato-feta mixture can be stored separately in airtight containers in the refrigerator for up to 3 days.

Variations and Tips:
- Use a variety of colored cherry tomatoes for a more vibrant presentation.
- Add diced cucumber or red onion to the tomato-feta mixture for extra flavor and crunch.
- Serve the grilled eggplant and tomato-feta mixture over a bed of mixed greens or with a side of whole grain bread for a more substantial meal.

Nutrition Facts:
Calories: 150 | Total Fat: 10g | Saturated Fat: 3g | Cholesterol: 15mg | Sodium: 350mg | Total Carbohydrates: 12g | Dietary Fiber: 4g | Total Sugars: 7g | Protein: 5g

This grilled eggplant with tomato and feta dish is an excellent choice for managing type 2 diabetes. Eggplant is a low-carb, fiber-rich vegetable, while the tomatoes and feta provide a flavorful and nutrient-dense topping. The dish is also low in calories and saturated fat, making it a healthy and satisfying option.

55. Beef and Vegetable Soup

Ingredients:
- 1 lb lean beef stew meat, cut into 1-inch cubes
- 2 tablespoons olive oil
- 1 onion, diced
- 3 cloves garlic, minced
- 4 cups low-sodium beef broth
- 1 (14.5 oz) can diced tomatoes
- 2 medium carrots, peeled and sliced
- 2 stalks celery, sliced
- 1 cup cubed potatoes
- 1 cup frozen green beans
- 1 teaspoon dried thyme
- 1 bay leaf
- Salt and black pepper to taste
- 2 tablespoons chopped fresh parsley (optional)

PreparationTime: 20 minutes

Cook Time: 1 hour 15 minutes

Total Time: 1 hour 35 minutes

Serves: 6

Directions:
1. In a large pot or Dutch oven, heat the olive oil over medium-high heat. Add the beef cubes and brown on all sides, about 5 minutes total. Remove the beef from the pot and set aside.
2. Add the onion and garlic to the pot and sauté for 2-3 minutes, until fragrant and translucent.
3. Pour in the beef broth and diced tomatoes, scraping up any browned bits from the bottom of the pot.
4. Add the browned beef, carrots, celery, potatoes, green beans, thyme, and bay leaf. Season with salt and black pepper to taste.
5. Bring the soup to a boil, then reduce the heat and simmer for 1 hour, or until the beef and vegetables are tender.
6. Remove the bay leaf. Stir in the chopped parsley, if using.
7. Serve the beef and vegetable soup hot.

Storage Instructions:
- Leftover soup can be stored in an airtight container in the refrigerator for up to 4 days or in the freezer for up to 3 months.

Variations and Tips:
- Use a combination of beef and ground turkey or chicken for a leaner protein source.
- Add other vegetables, such as zucchini, spinach, or mushrooms, to the soup.
- Serve the soup with a side of whole grain bread or crackers for a more filling meal.

Nutrition Facts:
Calories: 300 | Total Fat: 10g | Saturated Fat: 3g | Cholesterol: 60mg | Sodium: 450mg | Total Carbohydrates: 20g | Dietary Fiber: 5g | Total Sugars: 6g | Protein: 30g

Dinner Recipes for Balanced Nutrition

56. Baked Chicken Thighs with Sweet Potatoes

Ingredients:
- 8 bone-in, skin-on chicken thighs
- 2 medium sweet potatoes, peeled and cubed
- 1 red onion, sliced
- 2 tablespoons olive oil
- 1 teaspoon paprika
- 1 teaspoon garlic powder
- 1/2 teaspoon dried thyme
- 1/4 teaspoon salt
- 1/4 teaspoon black pepper

PreparationTime: 15 minutes
Cook Time: 45 minutes
Total Time: 1 hour
Serves: 4

Directions:
1. Preheat oven to 400°F. Line a large baking sheet with parchment paper or foil.

2. Place the chicken thighs, sweet potato cubes, and red onion slices on the prepared baking sheet. Drizzle with olive oil and sprinkle with paprika, garlic powder, dried thyme, salt, and black pepper. Toss to coat the ingredients evenly.

3. Bake for 40-45 minutes, or until the chicken is cooked through (internal temperature reaches 165°F) and the sweet potatoes are tender.

4. Serve the baked chicken thighs with the roasted sweet potatoes and onions.

Storage Instructions:
- Leftover chicken and sweet potatoes can be stored in an airtight container in the refrigerator for up to 3 days.

Variations and Tips:
- Use boneless, skinless chicken thighs or breasts for a leaner option.
- Add other vegetables, such as Brussels sprouts or green beans, to the baking sheet.
- Serve the chicken and sweet potatoes over a bed of quinoa or brown rice for a more complete meal.

Nutrition Facts:
Calories: 350 | Total Fat: 15g | Saturated Fat: 4g | Cholesterol: 120mg | Sodium: 350mg | Total Carbohydrates: 25g | Dietary Fiber: 5g | Total Sugars: 8g | Protein: 30g

This baked chicken thighs with sweet potatoes recipe is an excellent choice for managing type 2 diabetes. The chicken provides a lean protein source, while the sweet potatoes are a nutrient-dense carbohydrate that is high in fiber and vitamins. The dish is also relatively low in calories and sodium, making it a healthy and satisfying meal option.

Dinner Recipes for Balanced Nutrition

57. Roasted Cauliflower Tacos

Ingredients:
- 1 head of cauliflower, cut into florets
- 2 tablespoons olive oil
- 1 teaspoon chili powder
- 1/2 teaspoon cumin
- 1/4 teaspoon garlic powder
- 1/4 teaspoon salt
- 8 small whole wheat tortillas
- 1 cup shredded cabbage
- 1/2 cup diced tomatoes
- 1/4 cup crumbled feta cheese
- 2 tablespoons chopped fresh cilantro
- 1 lime, cut into wedges

PreparationTime: 20 minutes
Cook Time: 25 minutes
Total Time: 45 minutes
Serves: 4 (2 tacos per serving)

Directions:
1. Preheat oven to 400°F. Line a baking sheet with parchment paper.
2. In a large bowl, toss the cauliflower florets with olive oil, chili powder, cumin, garlic powder, and salt. Spread the seasoned cauliflower in a single layer on the prepared baking sheet.
3. Roast the cauliflower for 20-25 minutes, stirring halfway, until tender and lightly browned.
4. Warm the whole wheat tortillas according to package instructions.
5. To assemble the tacos, place a portion of the roasted cauliflower in each tortilla. Top with shredded cabbage, diced tomatoes, crumbled feta cheese, and chopped cilantro.
6. Serve the roasted cauliflower tacos with lime wedges for squeezing over the top.

Storage Instructions:
- Leftover roasted cauliflower can be stored in an airtight container in the refrigerator for up to 4 days.

Variations and Tips:
- Use a combination of roasted vegetables, such as sweet potatoes or bell peppers, in the tacos.
- Add a drizzle of Greek yogurt or avocado for extra creaminess.
- Serve the tacos with a side of black beans or a fresh salad for a more complete meal.

Nutrition Facts:
Calories: 250 | Total Fat: 10g | Saturated Fat: 2g | Cholesterol: 10mg | Sodium: 450mg | Total Carbohydrates: 30g | Dietary Fiber: 7g | Total Sugars: 5g | Protein: 10g

These roasted cauliflower tacos are an excellent choice for managing type 2 diabetes. Cauliflower is a low-carb, high-fiber vegetable that provides a satisfying and nutrient-dense base for the tacos. The whole wheat tortillas, cabbage, and tomatoes add additional fiber and vitamins, while the feta cheese provides a flavorful topping. This dish is a healthy and delicious option for those looking to manage their diabetes.

Dinner Recipes for Balanced Nutrition

58. Seared Scallops with Asparagus

Ingredients:
- 1 lb sea scallops, patted dry
- 2 tablespoons olive oil, divided
- 1 lb asparagus, trimmed and cut into 1-inch pieces
- 2 cloves garlic, minced
- 2 tablespoons lemon juice
- 2 tablespoons chopped fresh parsley
- Salt and black pepper to taste

PreparationTime: 15 minutes
Cook Time: 15 minutes
Total Time: 30 minutes
Serves: 4

Directions:

1. Heat 1 tablespoon of olive oil in a large skillet over medium-high heat.

2. Season the scallops with salt and black pepper. Sear the scallops for 2-3 minutes per side, until they are golden brown and cooked through. Remove the scallops from the skillet and set aside.

3. In the same skillet, heat the remaining 1 tablespoon of olive oil over medium heat. Add the asparagus and garlic, and sauté for 5-7 minutes, until the asparagus is tender-crisp.

4. Stir in the lemon juice and parsley. Season with additional salt and black pepper to taste.

5. Serve the seared scallops on top of the sautéed asparagus.

Storage Instructions:
- Leftover scallops and asparagus can be stored separately in airtight containers in the refrigerator for up to 2 days.

Variations and Tips:
- Use a combination of scallops and shrimp for added seafood flavor.
- Roast the asparagus in the oven instead of sautéing for a different texture.
- Serve the scallops and asparagus over a bed of quinoa or cauliflower rice for a more complete meal.

Nutrition Facts:
Calories: 200 | Total Fat: 8g | Saturated Fat: 1g | Cholesterol: 50mg | Sodium: 350mg | Total Carbohydrates: 10g | Dietary Fiber: 4g | Total Sugars: 3g | Protein: 22g

This seared scallops with asparagus dish is an excellent choice for managing type 2 diabetes. Scallops are a lean, high-protein seafood, while asparagus is a nutrient-dense vegetable that is low in carbohydrates. The simple preparation and use of healthy fats, such as olive oil, make this a balanced and diabetes-friendly meal.

59. Vegetable and Chicken Skewers

Ingredients:
- 1 lb boneless, skinless chicken breasts, cut into 1-inch cubes
- 1 red bell pepper, cut into 1-inch pieces
- 1 yellow bell pepper, cut into 1-inch pieces
- 1 zucchini, cut into 1-inch pieces
- 1 red onion, cut into 1-inch pieces
- 2 tablespoons olive oil
- 2 tablespoons balsamic vinegar
- 1 teaspoon dried oregano
- 1/2 teaspoon garlic powder
- 1/4 teaspoon salt
- 1/4 teaspoon black pepper

PreparationTime: 20 minutes
Cook Time: 15 minutes
Total Time: 35 minutes
Serves: 4

Directions:
1. Preheat grill or grill pan to medium-high heat.

2. In a large bowl, combine the chicken, bell peppers, zucchini, and onion. Drizzle with olive oil and balsamic vinegar, then sprinkle with oregano, garlic powder, salt, and black pepper. Toss to coat the ingredients evenly.

3. Thread the chicken and vegetables onto skewers, alternating the ingredients.

4. Grill the skewers for 12-15 minutes, turning occasionally, until the chicken is cooked through and the vegetables are tender. Serve the vegetable and chicken skewers immediately.

Storage Instructions:
- Leftover skewers can be stored in an airtight container in the refrigerator for up to 3 days.

Variations and Tips:
- Use different types of vegetables, such as mushrooms, cherry tomatoes, or eggplant.
- Marinate the chicken in the balsamic vinegar mixture for 30 minutes to 1 hour before assembling the skewers for more flavor.
- Soak wooden skewers in water for 30 minutes before using to prevent them from burning.
- Serve the skewers with a side of quinoa or a fresh salad for a complete meal.

Nutrition Facts:
Calories: 250 | Total Fat: 10g | Saturated Fat: 2g | Cholesterol: 70mg | Sodium: 300mg | Total Carbohydrates: 15g | Dietary Fiber: 4g | Total Sugars: 7g | Protein: 25g

This vegetable and chicken skewers recipe is an excellent choice for managing type 2 diabetes. The combination of lean protein from the chicken and fiber-rich vegetables provides a balanced and nutrient-dense meal. The use of healthy fats, such as olive oil, and the minimal seasoning keep the dish light and diabetes-friendly.

Dinner Recipes for Balanced Nutrition

60. Quinoa-Stuffed Bell Peppers

Ingredients:
- 4 bell peppers (any color)
- 1 cup quinoa, rinsed
- 2 cups vegetable or chicken broth
- 1 tablespoon olive oil
- 1 onion, diced
- 2 cloves garlic, minced
- 1 cup diced tomatoes
- 1 cup cooked black beans, rinsed and drained
- 1 teaspoon ground cumin
- 1 teaspoon dried oregano
- Salt and black pepper to taste
- 1/2 cup shredded cheddar or mozzarella cheese (optional)

PreparationTime: 20 minutes
Cook Time: 40 minutes
Total Time: 1 hour

Serves: 4

Directions:
1. Preheat the oven to 375°F (190°C).
2. Cut the tops off the bell peppers and remove the seeds and membranes. Place the peppers in a baking dish.
3. In a medium saucepan, combine the quinoa and broth. Bring to a boil, then reduce heat, cover, and simmer for 15-20 minutes, until the quinoa is cooked and the liquid is absorbed.
4. In a skillet, heat the olive oil over medium heat. Add the onion and garlic, and sauté for 2-3 minutes until fragrant.
5. Add the cooked quinoa, diced tomatoes, black beans, cumin, and oregano. Season with salt and black pepper to taste. Stir to combine.
6. Spoon the quinoa mixture into the hollowed-out bell peppers. Top with shredded cheese, if desired.
7. Bake for 30-40 minutes, or until the peppers are tender and the filling is hot.

Storage Instructions:
Leftover stuffed peppers can be stored in an airtight container in the refrigerator for up to 3-4 days. Reheat in the oven or microwave before serving.

Variations and Tips:
- Use different types of beans or grains, such as brown rice or farro, instead of quinoa.
- Add diced vegetables like zucchini, spinach, or mushrooms to the filling.
- Top the stuffed peppers with a dollop of Greek yogurt or a drizzle of balsamic glaze.
- For a spicier version, add diced jalapeño or red pepper flakes to the filling.

Nutrition Facts:
Calories: 250 - Total Fat: 7g - Saturated Fat: 2g - Cholesterol: 10mg
Sodium: 450mg - Total Carbohydrates: 37g - Dietary Fiber: 8g - Sugars: 6g - Protein: 11g

Dinner Recipes for Balanced Nutrition

61. Apple Slices with Almond Butter

Ingredients:
- 1 medium apple, sliced
- 2 tablespoons almond butter

PreparationTime: 5 minutes
Cook Time: 0 minutes
Total Time: 5 minutes

Directions:

1. Wash and slice the apple into thin wedges.

Serves: 1

2. Spread the almond butter evenly over the apple slices.

Storage Instructions:

This snack is best enjoyed immediately, but any leftover apple slices can be stored in an airtight container in the refrigerator for up to 3 days.

Variations and Tips:

- Use different types of nut butters, such as peanut butter or cashew butter, if preferred.

- Sprinkle a pinch of cinnamon over the apple slices for added flavor.

- For a crunchier texture, top the almond butter with chopped nuts or granola.

Nutrition Facts:

Calories: 150
Total Fat: 10g
Saturated Fat: 1g
Cholesterol: 0mg
Sodium: 0mg
Total Carbohydrates: 15g
Dietary Fiber: 4g
Sugars: 11g
Protein: 4g

This snack is an excellent choice for managing type 2 diabetes. The combination of the apple's natural sweetness and the healthy fats and protein from the almond butter helps to keep blood sugar levels stable. The fiber in the apple also helps to slow the absorption of carbohydrates, further supporting blood sugar management.

Snack Ideas to Keep Blood Sugar Stable

62. Carrot Sticks with Hummus

Ingredients:
- 1 medium carrot, peeled and cut into sticks
- 2 tablespoons hummus

PreparationTime: 10 minutes
Cook Time: 0 minutes
Total Time: 10 minutes

Serves: 1

Directions:
1. Wash and peel the carrot, then cut it into thin, long sticks.
2. Serve the carrot sticks with the hummus for dipping.

Storage Instructions:
The carrot sticks and hummus can be stored separately in airtight containers in the refrigerator for up to 3-4 days.

Variations and Tips:
- Try different flavors of hummus, such as roasted red pepper or garlic, for variety.
- Add a sprinkle of paprika or cayenne pepper to the hummus for a little kick.
- Serve the carrot sticks with other crunchy vegetables, like celery or cucumber, for a more varied snack.

Nutrition Facts:
Calories: 80
Total Fat: 4g
Saturated Fat: 0g
Cholesterol: 0mg
Sodium: 160mg
Total Carbohydrates: 10g
Dietary Fiber: 3g
Sugars: 5g
Protein: 3g

This snack is an excellent choice for managing type 2 diabetes. The carrot sticks provide a crunchy, low-calorie, and low-carbohydrate vegetable, while the hummus adds a source of healthy fats and protein to help keep blood sugar levels stable. The fiber in the carrot and the complex carbohydrates in the hummus also help to slow the absorption of carbohydrates, further supporting blood sugar management.

Snack Ideas to Keep Blood Sugar Stable

63. Greek Yogurt with Cucumber Slices

Ingredients:
- 1/2 cup plain Greek yogurt
- 1/2 medium cucumber, sliced

PreparationTime: 5 minutes

Cook Time: 0 minutes

Total Time: 5 minutes

Serves: 1

Directions:
1. Scoop the Greek yogurt into a small bowl.

2. Arrange the cucumber slices around the yogurt.

Storage Instructions:
The yogurt and cucumber can be stored separately in airtight containers in the refrigerator for up to 3-4 days.

Variations and Tips:
- Top the yogurt with a sprinkle of chopped fresh herbs, such as dill or mint, for added flavor.

- Drizzle a small amount of honey or a squeeze of lemon juice over the yogurt for a touch of sweetness.

- Serve the cucumber slices with other crunchy vegetables, like bell pepper or carrot sticks, for a more varied snack.

Nutrition Facts:
Calories: 100
Total Fat: 3g
Saturated Fat: 2g
Cholesterol: 15mg
Sodium: 45mg
Total Carbohydrates: 8g
Dietary Fiber: 1g
Sugars: 8g
Protein: 12g

This snack is an excellent choice for managing type 2 diabetes. The Greek yogurt provides a good source of protein, which helps to keep blood sugar levels stable. The cucumber slices are a low-calorie, low-carbohydrate vegetable that adds crunch and hydration. The combination of the protein-rich yogurt and the fiber-rich cucumber makes this a well-balanced snack that can help manage blood sugar levels.

64. Mixed Nuts and Seeds

Ingredients:
- 1/4 cup mixed nuts (such as almonds,
  walnuts, cashews, and pecans)
- 1 tablespoon mixed seeds (such as pumpkin,
sunflower, and chia seeds)

PreparationTime: 5 minutes

Cook Time: 0 minutes

Total Time: 5 minutes

Serves: 1

Directions:
1. Combine the mixed nuts and seeds in a small bowl or resealable bag.

Storage Instructions:
The mixed nuts and seeds can be stored in an airtight container or resealable bag at room temperature for up to 2 weeks.

Variations and Tips:

- Roast the nuts and seeds lightly for added crunch and flavor.

- Add a sprinkle of cinnamon or a pinch of sea salt for extra seasoning.

- Mix in a few dried berries or dark chocolate chips for a touch of sweetness.

- Portion the nuts and seeds into individual servings for easy grab-and-go snacks.

Nutrition Facts:
Calories: 200
Total Fat: 18g
Saturated Fat: 2g
Cholesterol: 0mg
Sodium: 0mg
Total Carbohydrates: 6g
Dietary Fiber: 3g
Sugars: 1g
Protein: 6g

This snack is an excellent choice for managing type 2 diabetes. The combination of nuts and seeds provides a good source of healthy fats, protein, and fiber, which can help to keep blood sugar levels stable. The fiber and healthy fats also help to promote feelings of fullness, which can prevent overeating and support weight management. Additionally, the variety of nuts and seeds offers a range of essential vitamins, minerals, and antioxidants that are beneficial for overall health.

Snack Ideas to Keep Blood Sugar Stable

65. Edamame with Sea Salt

Ingredients:
- 1 cup frozen edamame, in the pod
- 1/4 teaspoon sea salt

PreparationTime: 5 minutes
Cook Time: 5 minutes
Total Time: 10 minutes

Serves: 1

Directions:
1. Bring a small pot of water to a boil.

2. Add the frozen edamame and cook for 5 minutes, or until tender.

3. Drain the edamame and sprinkle with sea salt.

Storage Instructions:
Cooked edamame can be stored in an airtight container in the refrigerator for up to 3-4 days.

Variations and Tips:

- Try different seasonings, such as garlic powder, chili powder, or lemon pepper, for added flavor.

- Serve the edamame warm or at room temperature.

- For a heartier snack, pair the edamame with a small handful of nuts or seeds.

Nutrition Facts:
Calories: 120
Total Fat: 5g
Saturated Fat: 0g
Cholesterol: 0mg
Sodium: 180mg
Total Carbohydrates: 9g
Dietary Fiber: 5g
Sugars: 2g
Protein: 11g

Edamame is an excellent snack choice for managing type 2 diabetes. The soybeans are a good source of plant-based protein, fiber, and complex carbohydrates, which can help to keep blood sugar levels stable. The fiber in edamame also helps to slow the absorption of carbohydrates, further supporting blood sugar management. Additionally, edamame is low in calories and contains no added sugars, making it a nutritious and satisfying snack option.

Snack Ideas to Keep Blood Sugar Stable

66. Cottage Cheese with Pineapple Chunks

Ingredients:
- 1/2 cup low-fat or non-fat cottage cheese
- 1/2 cup fresh pineapple chunks

PreparationTime: 5 minutes
Cook Time: 0 minutes
Total Time: 5 minutes

Directions:
1. Scoop the cottage cheese into a small bowl.

Serves: 1

2. Top the cottage cheese with the pineapple chunks.

Storage Instructions:
The cottage cheese and pineapple can be stored separately in airtight containers in the refrigerator for up to 3-4 days.

Variations and Tips:
- Try different types of fruit, such as berries, melon, or kiwi, instead of pineapple.
- Sprinkle a small amount of cinnamon or a drizzle of honey over the cottage cheese for added flavor.
- For a creamier texture, blend the cottage cheese with a splash of milk or yogurt before adding the fruit.

Nutrition Facts:
Calories: 150
Total Fat: 3g
Saturated Fat: 2g
Cholesterol: 15mg
Sodium: 300mg
Total Carbohydrates: 15g
Dietary Fiber: 2g
Sugars: 12g
Protein: 15g

This snack is an excellent choice for managing type 2 diabetes. The cottage cheese provides a good source of protein, which can help to keep blood sugar levels stable. The pineapple chunks add natural sweetness and fiber, which can help to slow the absorption of carbohydrates. The combination of the protein-rich cottage cheese and the fiber-rich pineapple makes this a well-balanced snack that can support blood sugar management.

Snack Ideas to Keep Blood Sugar Stable

67. Cherry Tomatoes with Mozzarella Balls

Ingredients:
- 10-12 cherry tomatoes, halved
- 1/4 cup fresh mozzarella balls (or cubed mozzarella)
- 1 teaspoon balsamic glaze (optional)
- Fresh basil leaves (optional)

PreparationTime: 5 minutes

Cook Time: 0 minutes

Total Time: 5 minutes

Serves: 1

Directions:

1. Arrange the halved cherry tomatoes and mozzarella balls on a small plate.

2. Drizzle the balsamic glaze over the top, if using.

3. Garnish with fresh basil leaves, if desired.

Storage Instructions:
The tomatoes and mozzarella can be stored separately in airtight containers in the refrigerator for up to 3-4 days.

Variations and Tips:
- Use different types of tomatoes, such as grape or heirloom, for variety.
- Substitute the mozzarella with cubes of feta or goat cheese.
- Add a sprinkle of dried Italian seasoning or a pinch of salt and pepper for extra flavor.
- Serve the tomatoes and mozzarella on toothpicks or skewers for a fun, portable snack.

Nutrition Facts:
Calories: 100
Total Fat: 6g
Saturated Fat: 3g
Cholesterol: 15mg
Sodium: 150mg
Total Carbohydrates: 6g
Dietary Fiber: 1g
Sugars: 4g
Protein: 7g

This snack is an excellent choice for managing type 2 diabetes. The cherry tomatoes are a low-calorie, low-carbohydrate vegetable that provides fiber and antioxidants. The mozzarella cheese adds a good source of protein, which can help to keep blood sugar levels stable. The combination of the fiber-rich tomatoes and the protein-rich cheese makes this a well-balanced snack that can support blood sugar management.

Snack Ideas to Keep Blood Sugar Stable

68. Hard-Boiled Eggs

Ingredients:
- 4 large eggs

PreparationTime: 15 minutes
Cook Time: 12 minutes
Total Time: 27 minutes

Serves: 2 (2 eggs per serving)

Directions:
1. Place the eggs in a single layer in a saucepan
and cover with cold water by 1 inch.

2. Bring the water to a boil over high heat.

3. Once the water is boiling, remove the pan
from the heat, cover, and let the eggs sit for 12 minutes.

4. Drain the hot water and cover the eggs with cold water to cool them down.

5. Peel the eggs and enjoy as a snack or use in other recipes.

Storage Instructions:
Hard-boiled eggs can be stored in the refrigerator, in their shells, for up to 1 week.

Variations and Tips:
- Season the hard-boiled eggs with a sprinkle of salt, pepper, or paprika for added flavor.

- Slice the eggs and serve them on a bed of greens or with a small amount of hummus or avocado for a more substantial snack.

- For a portable snack, pack the hard-boiled eggs in a small container or resealable bag.

Nutrition Facts:
Calories: 140
Total Fat: 10g
Saturated Fat: 3g
Cholesterol: 375mg
Sodium: 70mg
Total Carbohydrates: 0g
Dietary Fiber: 0g
Sugars: 0g
Protein: 12g

Hard-boiled eggs are an excellent snack choice for managing type 2 diabetes. They are a good source of high-quality protein, which can help to keep blood sugar levels stable. Eggs also contain no carbohydrates, making them a low-impact food for individuals with diabetes. Additionally, the protein in eggs can help to promote feelings of fullness, which can prevent overeating and support weight management.

Snack Ideas to Keep Blood Sugar Stable

69. Celery Sticks with Peanut Butter

Ingredients:
- 2-3 celery stalks, cut into 3-inch sticks
- 2 tablespoons natural peanut butter

PreparationTime: 5 minutes
Cook Time: 0 minutes
Total Time: 5 minutes

Serves: 1

Directions:
1. Wash and cut the celery stalks into 3-inch sticks.

2. Spread the peanut butter evenly over the celery sticks.

Storage Instructions:

The celery sticks and peanut butter can be stored separately in airtight containers in the refrigerator for up to 3-4 days.

Variations and Tips:

- Use different nut butters, such as almond or cashew butter, for variety.
- Sprinkle a pinch of cinnamon or a drizzle of honey over the peanut butter for added flavor.
- For a crunchier texture, top the peanut butter with chopped nuts or seeds.

Nutrition Facts:

Calories: 150
Total Fat: 10g
Saturated Fat: 2g
Cholesterol: 0mg
Sodium: 150mg
Total Carbohydrates: 10g
Dietary Fiber: 3g
Sugars: 4g
Protein: 6g

This snack is an excellent choice for managing type 2 diabetes. The celery sticks provide a crunchy, low-calorie, and low-carbohydrate vegetable, while the peanut butter adds a good source of healthy fats and protein to help keep blood sugar levels stable. The fiber in the celery and the complex carbohydrates in the peanut butter also help to slow the absorption of carbohydrates, further supporting blood sugar management.

Snack Ideas to Keep Blood Sugar Stable

70. Roasted Chickpeas with Spices

Ingredients:
- 1 (15-ounce) can chickpeas, rinsed and drained
- 1 tablespoon olive oil
- 1 teaspoon ground cumin
- 1 teaspoon paprika
- 1/4 teaspoon garlic powder
- 1/4 teaspoon salt

PreparationTime: 10 minutes
Cook Time: 25 minutes
Total Time: 35 minutes

Serves: 2 (1/2 cup per serving)

Directions:
1. Preheat the oven to 400°F (200°C).

2. Pat the chickpeas dry with a paper towel to remove any excess moisture.

3. In a small bowl, toss the chickpeas with the olive oil, cumin, paprika, garlic powder, and salt until evenly coated.

4. Spread the chickpeas in a single layer on a baking sheet.

5. Roast for 20-25 minutes, stirring halfway, until the chickpeas are crispy.

6. Allow the roasted chickpeas to cool slightly before serving.

Storage Instructions: The roasted chickpeas can be stored in an airtight container at room temperature for up to 5 days.

Variations and Tips:
- Experiment with different spice blends, such as chili powder, curry powder, or Italian seasoning.
- For a sweeter version, toss the roasted chickpeas with a small amount of honey or maple syrup.
- Add a sprinkle of grated Parmesan cheese or chopped fresh herbs for extra flavor.

Nutrition Facts:
Calories: 150 - Total Fat: 6g - Saturated Fat: 1g - Cholesterol: 0mg - Sodium: 300mg
Total Carbohydrates: 18g - Dietary Fiber: 5g - Sugars: 2g - Protein: 6g

Roasted chickpeas are an excellent snack choice for managing type 2 diabetes. Chickpeas are a good source of complex carbohydrates, fiber, and protein, which can help to keep blood sugar levels stable. The roasting process also helps to reduce the glycemic index of the chickpeas, further supporting blood sugar management. Additionally, the spices used in this recipe add flavor without adding any extra carbohydrates or sugars.

Snack Ideas to Keep Blood Sugar Stable

71. Whole Grain Crackers with Avocado

Ingredients:
- 4-5 whole grain crackers
- 1/2 medium avocado, mashed

PreparationTime: 5 minutes
Cook Time: 0 minutes
Total Time: 5 minutes

Directions:
1. Spread the mashed avocado evenly over the whole grain crackers.

Serves: 1

Storage Instructions:
The avocado can be stored in an airtight container in the refrigerator for up to 3 days. The crackers can be stored in their original packaging at room temperature.

Variations and Tips:

- Top the avocado with a sprinkle of salt, pepper, or a squeeze of lemon juice for added flavor.

- For a creamier texture, mix the mashed avocado with a small amount of plain Greek yogurt.

- Use different types of whole grain crackers, such as rye, whole wheat, or multigrain, for variety.

- Add a few slices of tomato or a sprinkle of chopped fresh herbs for extra nutrition and flavor.

Nutrition Facts:
Calories: 200
Total Fat: 13g
Saturated Fat: 2g
Cholesterol: 0mg
Sodium: 150mg
Total Carbohydrates: 18g
Dietary Fiber: 6g
Sugars: 1g
Protein: 4g

This snack is an excellent choice for managing type 2 diabetes. The whole grain crackers provide complex carbohydrates and fiber, which can help to slow the absorption of carbohydrates and keep blood sugar levels stable. The avocado adds healthy fats and a creamy texture, which can also help to promote feelings of fullness and prevent overeating. The combination of the fiber-rich crackers and the healthy fats from the avocado makes this a well-balanced snack that can support blood sugar management.

Snack Ideas to Keep Blood Sugar Stable

72. Bell Pepper Slices with Guacamole

Ingredients:
- 1 medium bell pepper, sliced into strips
- 2 tablespoons homemade or store-bought guacamole

PreparationTime: 10 minutes
Cook Time: 0 minutes
Total Time: 10 minutes

Serves: 1

Directions:
1. Wash and slice the bell pepper into thin, long strips.

2. Serve the bell pepper slices with the guacamole for dipping.

Storage Instructions:
The bell pepper slices and guacamole can be stored separately in airtight containers in the refrigerator for up to 3-4 days.

Variations and Tips:

- Use a variety of bell pepper colors, such as red, yellow, and orange, for a more visually appealing snack.

- Add a sprinkle of chili powder or a squeeze of lime juice to the guacamole for extra flavor.

- Serve the bell pepper and guacamole with a small handful of raw nuts or seeds for a more substantial snack.

Nutrition Facts:
Calories: 100
Total Fat: 7g
Saturated Fat: 1g
Cholesterol: 0mg
Sodium: 150mg
Total Carbohydrates: 8g
Dietary Fiber: 4g
Sugars: 4g
Protein: 2g

This snack is an excellent choice for managing type 2 diabetes. The bell pepper slices are a low-calorie, low-carbohydrate vegetable that provides fiber and essential vitamins and minerals. The guacamole adds healthy fats from the avocado, which can help to slow the absorption of carbohydrates and keep blood sugar levels stable. The combination of the fiber-rich bell pepper and the healthy fats from the guacamole makes this a well-balanced snack that can support blood sugar management.

73. Cucumber Slices with Tzatziki

Ingredients:
- 1 medium cucumber, sliced
- 2 tablespoons homemade or store-bought tzatziki sauce

PreparationTime: 10 minutes
Cook Time: 0 minutes
Total Time: 10 minutes

Serves: 1

Directions:
1. Wash and slice the cucumber into thin, round slices.

2. Serve the cucumber slices with the tzatziki sauce for dipping.

Storage Instructions:
The cucumber slices and tzatziki sauce can be stored separately in airtight containers in the refrigerator for up to 3-4 days.

Variations and Tips:

- Try using different types of cucumbers, such as English or Persian, for variety.

- Add a sprinkle of dill, lemon zest, or a pinch of garlic powder to the tzatziki for extra flavor.

- Serve the cucumber and tzatziki with a small handful of roasted chickpeas or a few olives for a more substantial snack.

Nutrition Facts:
Calories: 80
Total Fat: 4g
Saturated Fat: 1g
Cholesterol: 5mg
Sodium: 150mg
Total Carbohydrates: 8g
Dietary Fiber: 2g
Sugars: 4g
Protein: 3g

This snack is an excellent choice for managing type 2 diabetes. The cucumber slices are a low-calorie, low-carbohydrate vegetable that provides hydration and fiber. The tzatziki sauce, made with Greek yogurt, adds a good source of protein, which can help to keep blood sugar levels stable. The combination of the fiber-rich cucumber and the protein-rich tzatziki makes this a well-balanced snack that can support blood sugar management.

Snack Ideas to Keep Blood Sugar Stable

74. Sliced Pear with Ricotta Cheese

Ingredients:
- 1 medium pear, sliced
- 2 tablespoons low-fat or part-skim ricotta cheese

PreparationTime: 5 minutes
Cook Time: 0 minutes
Total Time: 5 minutes

Serves: 1

Directions:
1. Wash and slice the pear into thin wedges.

2. Arrange the pear slices on a plate and top with the ricotta cheese.

Storage Instructions:
The sliced pear and ricotta cheese can be stored separately in airtight containers in the refrigerator for up to 3-4 days.

Variations and Tips:
- Sprinkle a small amount of cinnamon or a drizzle of honey over the ricotta cheese for added flavor.

- Use different types of pears, such as Bartlett or Bosc, for variety.

- Serve the pear and ricotta with a small handful of chopped nuts or a few whole grain crackers for a more substantial snack.

Nutrition Facts:

Calories: 150
Total Fat: 5g
Saturated Fat: 3g
Cholesterol: 20mg
Sodium: 70mg
Total Carbohydrates: 20g
Dietary Fiber: 4g
Sugars: 12g
Protein: 7g

This snack is an excellent choice for managing type 2 diabetes. The pear provides natural sweetness and fiber, which can help to slow the absorption of carbohydrates and keep blood sugar levels stable. The ricotta cheese adds a good source of protein, which can also help to regulate blood sugar. The combination of the fiber-rich pear and the protein-rich ricotta makes this a well-balanced snack that can support blood sugar management.

Snack Ideas to Keep Blood Sugar Stable

75. Almonds with Dark Chocolate Chips

Ingredients:
- 1/4 cup raw, unsalted almonds
- 1 tablespoon dark chocolate chips

PreparationTime: 5 minutes
Cook Time: 0 minutes
Total Time: 5 minutes

Directions:
1. Combine the almonds and dark chocolate chips in a small bowl or resealable bag.

Serves: 1

Storage Instructions:
The almond and dark chocolate chip mixture can be stored in an airtight container at room temperature for up to 1 week.

Variations and Tips:
- Use a higher percentage of dark chocolate (70% or more) for a richer, less sweet flavor.

- Add a sprinkle of sea salt or a pinch of cinnamon to the mixture for extra flavor.

- Substitute the dark chocolate chips with a small amount of unsweetened shredded coconut or chopped nuts, such as pecans or walnuts.

Nutrition Facts:

Calories: 200
Total Fat: 16g
Saturated Fat: 3g
Cholesterol: 0mg
Sodium: 0mg
Total Carbohydrates: 10g
Dietary Fiber: 4g
Sugars: 5g
Protein: 6g

This snack is an excellent choice for managing type 2 diabetes. Almonds are a good source of healthy fats, protein, and fiber, which can help to keep blood sugar levels stable. The dark chocolate chips provide a small amount of carbohydrates and antioxidants, while also satisfying a sweet craving. The combination of the healthy fats, protein, and fiber from the almonds, along with the moderation of the dark chocolate, makes this a well-balanced snack that can support blood sugar management.

Snack Ideas to Keep Blood Sugar Stable

76. Sliced Turkey Roll-Ups with Spinach

Ingredients:
- 2-3 slices of deli-style turkey breast
- 1/2 cup fresh spinach leaves
- 1 teaspoon Dijon mustard (optional)

PreparationTime: 5 minutes
Cook Time: 0 minutes
Total Time: 5 minutes

Serves: 1

Directions:
1. Lay the turkey slices flat on a clean surface.

2. Place the spinach leaves on top of the turkey slices.

3. If using, spread a small amount of Dijon mustard over the spinach.

4. Carefully roll up the turkey slices, enclosing the spinach inside.

Storage Instructions:
The turkey roll-ups can be stored in an airtight container in the refrigerator for up to 3-4 days.

Variations and Tips:
- Use different types of deli meat, such as roast beef or ham, for variety.
- Add a thin slice of cheese, such as cheddar or Swiss, to the roll-ups for extra flavor and protein.
- Serve the turkey roll-ups with a small side of cherry tomatoes or cucumber slices for a more complete snack.

Nutrition Facts:

Calories: 100
Total Fat: 2g
Saturated Fat: 0g
Cholesterol: 30mg
Sodium: 450mg
Total Carbohydrates: 2g
Dietary Fiber: 1g
Sugars: 1g
Protein: 16g

This snack is an excellent choice for managing type 2 diabetes. The turkey provides a good source of lean protein, which can help to keep blood sugar levels stable. The spinach adds fiber, vitamins, and minerals, while also providing a low-carbohydrate vegetable. The combination of the protein-rich turkey and the fiber-rich spinach makes this a well-balanced snack that can support blood sugar management.

Snack Ideas to Keep Blood Sugar Stable

77. Mixed Berry Parfait with Greek Yogurt

Ingredients:
- 1/2 cup mixed berries
(such as blueberries, raspberries, and blackberries)
- 1/2 cup plain Greek yogurt
- 1 teaspoon honey (optional)

PreparationTime: 10 minutes
Cook Time: 0 minutes
Total Time: 10 minutes

Serves: 1

Directions:

1. Layer the mixed berries and Greek yogurt in a small glass or bowl.

2. If desired, drizzle a small amount of honey over the top.

Storage Instructions:

The parfait can be stored in an airtight container in the refrigerator for up to 3-4 days.

Variations and Tips:

- Use different types of berries, such as strawberries or cranberries, for variety.

- Sprinkle a small amount of chopped nuts, such as almonds or walnuts, over the top for added crunch and healthy fats.

- For a creamier texture, blend the Greek yogurt with a splash of milk or a bit of vanilla extract before layering with the berries.

Nutrition Facts:

Calories: 150
Total Fat: 3g
Saturated Fat: 1g
Cholesterol: 10mg
Sodium: 45mg
Total Carbohydrates: 20g
Dietary Fiber: 4g
Sugars: 14g
Protein: 12g

This snack is an excellent choice for managing type 2 diabetes. The mixed berries provide natural sweetness and fiber, which can help to slow the absorption of carbohydrates and keep blood sugar levels stable. The Greek yogurt adds a good source of protein, which can also help to regulate blood sugar. The combination of the fiber-rich berries and the protein-rich yogurt makes this a well-balanced snack that can support blood sugar management.

Snack Ideas to Keep Blood Sugar Stable

78. Sliced Kiwi with Cottage Cheese

Ingredients:
- 1 medium kiwi, peeled and sliced
- 1/2 cup low-fat or non-fat cottage cheese

PreparationTime: 5 minutes
Cook Time: 0 minutes
Total Time: 5 minutes

Serves: 1

Directions:

1. Arrange the sliced kiwi on a plate or in a small bowl.

2. Top the kiwi slices with the cottage cheese.

Storage Instructions:

The sliced kiwi and cottage cheese can be stored separately in airtight containers in the refrigerator for up to 3-4 days.

Variations and Tips:

- Sprinkle a small amount of cinnamon or a drizzle of honey over the cottage cheese for added flavor.

- Use different types of fruit, such as berries or melon, instead of kiwi.

- Serve the kiwi and cottage cheese with a small handful of chopped nuts or seeds for a more substantial snack.

Nutrition Facts:

Calories: 150
Total Fat: 3g
Saturated Fat: 1g
Cholesterol: 10mg
Sodium: 300mg
Total Carbohydrates: 15g
Dietary Fiber: 3g
Sugars: 10g
Protein: 15g

This snack is an excellent choice for managing type 2 diabetes. The kiwi provides natural sweetness, fiber, and a good source of vitamin C, while the cottage cheese adds a good source of protein. The combination of the fiber-rich kiwi and the protein-rich cottage cheese makes this a well-balanced snack that can help to keep blood sugar levels stable. Additionally, the low-fat or non-fat cottage cheese is a low-calorie, low-carbohydrate option that can support weight management.

Snack Ideas to Keep Blood Sugar Stable

79. Sliced Mango with Chili Powder

Ingredients:
- 1 medium mango, peeled and sliced
- 1/4 teaspoon chili powder

PreparationTime: 5 minutes
Cook Time: 0 minutes
Total Time: 5 minutes

Serves: 1

Directions:
1. Arrange the sliced mango on a plate or in a small bowl.

2. Sprinkle the chili powder evenly over the mango slices.

Storage Instructions:
The sliced mango can be stored in an airtight container in the refrigerator for up to 3-4 days.

Variations and Tips:

- Use a combination of chili powder and a small amount of lime juice or zest for a tangy-spicy flavor.
- Experiment with different spices, such as cayenne pepper, cumin, or paprika, for a variety of flavors.
- Serve the mango slices with a small handful of roasted unsalted nuts for a more substantial snack.

Nutrition Facts:

Calories: 100
Total Fat: 0g
Saturated Fat: 0g
Cholesterol: 0mg
Sodium: 0mg
Total Carbohydrates: 25g
Dietary Fiber: 3g
Sugars: 20g
Protein: 1g

This snack is an excellent choice for managing type 2 diabetes. Mango is a sweet, low-glycemic fruit that provides fiber, vitamins, and minerals. The chili powder adds a spicy kick without adding any extra carbohydrates or sugars. The combination of the natural sweetness from the mango and the heat from the chili powder can help to satisfy cravings for something sweet and flavorful, while the fiber in the mango can help to slow the absorption of carbohydrates and keep blood sugar levels stable.

Snack Ideas to Keep Blood Sugar Stable

80. Blueberry Smoothie with Spinach and Protein Powder

Ingredients:
- 1 cup fresh or frozen blueberries
- 1 cup unsweetened almond milk (or milk of your choice)
- 1 cup fresh spinach leaves
- 1 scoop vanilla or unflavored protein powder
- 1 tablespoon ground flaxseed (optional)
- Ice cubes (optional)

PreparationTime: 5 minutes
Cook Time: 0 minutes
Total Time: 5 minutes

Serves: 1

Directions:
1. Add all the ingredients to a high-speed blender and blend until smooth and creamy.

2. If desired, add a few ice cubes and blend again to chill the smoothie.

Storage Instructions: The smoothie can be stored in an airtight container in the refrigerator for up to 1 day.

Variations and Tips:

- Use different types of berries, such as raspberries or blackberries, instead of blueberries.
- Add a small amount of peanut butter or almond butter for extra protein and healthy fats.
- Substitute the protein powder with Greek yogurt for a creamier texture.
- Sprinkle a small amount of cinnamon or nutmeg over the top for added flavor.

Nutrition Facts:

Calories: 200
Total Fat: 5g
Saturated Fat: 0g
Cholesterol: 0mg
Sodium: 150mg
Total Carbohydrates: 25g
Dietary Fiber: 6g
Sugars: 15g
Protein: 15g

This smoothie is an excellent choice for managing type 2 diabetes. The blueberries provide natural sweetness and fiber, which can help to slow the absorption of carbohydrates and keep blood sugar levels stable. The spinach adds a boost of vitamins, minerals, and fiber, while the protein powder helps to provide a sustained source of energy and support muscle maintenance. The combination of the fiber-rich fruits and vegetables, the protein from the powder, and the healthy fats from the optional nut butter or yogurt makes this a well-balanced snack that can support blood sugar management.

Snack Ideas to Keep Blood Sugar Stable

81. Baked Apple with Cinnamon

Ingredients:
- 1 medium apple, cored and sliced
- 1 teaspoon ground cinnamon
- 1 tablespoon water

PreparationTime: 10 minutes
Cook Time: 20 minutes
Total Time: 30 minutes

Serves: 1

Directions:

1. Preheat the oven to 375°F (190°C).

2. Place the apple slices in a small baking dish and sprinkle with the ground cinnamon.

3. Pour the water into the baking dish.

4. Bake for 20-25 minutes, or until the apples are tender and fragrant.

Storage Instructions:

The baked apples can be stored in an airtight container in the refrigerator for up to 3-4 days.

Variations and Tips:

- Use a variety of apples, such as Gala, Honeycrisp, or Fuji, for different flavors and textures.
- Add a sprinkle of nutmeg or a drizzle of lemon juice for extra flavor.
- Serve the baked apples with a small dollop of plain Greek yogurt or a sprinkle of chopped nuts for a more substantial snack.

Nutrition Facts:

Calories: 80
Total Fat: 0g
Saturated Fat: 0g
Cholesterol: 0mg
Sodium: 0mg
Total Carbohydrates: 20g
Dietary Fiber: 3g
Sugars: 15g
Protein: 0g

This snack is an excellent choice for managing type 2 diabetes. Apples are a low-glycemic fruit that provide fiber, which can help to slow the absorption of carbohydrates and keep blood sugar levels stable. The cinnamon adds flavor without any extra carbohydrates or sugars. The baking process also helps to concentrate the natural sweetness of the apples, making this a satisfying and healthy snack option for individuals with type 2 diabetes.

Desserts that Won't Spike Your Blood Sugar

82. Greek Yogurt with Honey and Walnuts

Ingredients:
- 1 cup plain Greek yogurt
- 1 teaspoon honey
- 2 tablespoons chopped walnuts

PreparationTime: 5 minutes
Cook Time: 0 minutes
Total Time: 5 minutes

Serves: 1

Directions:

1. Scoop the Greek yogurt into a small bowl.

2. Drizzle the honey over the yogurt.

3. Sprinkle the chopped walnuts on top.

Storage Instructions:

The Greek yogurt, honey, and walnuts can be stored separately in airtight containers in the refrigerator for up to 3-4 days.

Variations and Tips:

- Use different types of nuts, such as almonds or pecans, instead of walnuts.
- Add a sprinkle of cinnamon or a squeeze of lemon juice for extra flavor.
- For a creamier texture, blend the Greek yogurt with a small amount of milk or unsweetened almond milk before adding the honey and nuts.

Nutrition Facts:

Calories: 200
Total Fat: 10g
Saturated Fat: 2g
Cholesterol: 20mg
Sodium: 65mg
Total Carbohydrates: 15g
Dietary Fiber: 2g
Sugars: 12g
Protein: 15g

This snack is an excellent choice for managing type 2 diabetes. The Greek yogurt provides a good source of protein, which can help to keep blood sugar levels stable. The honey adds a touch of natural sweetness, while the walnuts provide healthy fats and a crunchy texture. The combination of the protein-rich yogurt, the fiber-rich nuts, and the moderate amount of natural sweetener makes this a well-balanced snack that can support blood sugar management.

Desserts that Won't Spike Your Blood Sugar

83. Chia Seed Pudding with Coconut Milk

Ingredients:
- 2 tablespoons chia seeds
- 1/2 cup unsweetened coconut milk
- 1 teaspoon vanilla extract
- 1/2 teaspoon ground cinnamon (optional)
- 1 tablespoon unsweetened shredded coconut (optional)

PreparationTime: 10 minutes
Cook Time: 0 minutes (chilling time: 2 hours)
Total Time: 2 hours 10 minutes

Serves: 1

Directions:

1. In a small bowl or jar, combine the chia seeds, coconut milk, and vanilla extract. Stir well to combine.

2. Cover and refrigerate for at least 2 hours, or until the chia seeds have thickened the mixture into a pudding-like consistency.

3. Sprinkle the ground cinnamon and shredded coconut (if using) over the top before serving.

Storage Instructions:

The chia seed pudding can be stored in an airtight container in the refrigerator for up to 3-4 days.

Variations and Tips:

- Use different types of milk, such as almond milk or unsweetened soy milk, instead of coconut milk.
- Add a small amount of fresh or frozen berries for extra flavor and nutrients.
- Drizzle a teaspoon of honey or maple syrup over the top for a touch of sweetness.

Nutrition Facts:

, Calories: 200 - Total Fat: 14g - Saturated Fat: 10g
Cholesterol: 0mg - Sodium: 20mg - Total Carbohydrates: 14g
Dietary Fiber: 8g - Sugars: 4g - Protein: 5g

This snack is an excellent choice for managing type 2 diabetes. Chia seeds are a good source of fiber, which can help to slow the absorption of carbohydrates and keep blood sugar levels stable. The coconut milk provides healthy fats, which can also help to regulate blood sugar. The combination of the fiber-rich chia seeds and the healthy fats from the coconut milk makes this a well-balanced snack that can support blood sugar management.

Desserts that Won't Spike Your Blood Sugar

84. Dark Chocolate and Almond Clusters

Ingredients:
- 1/2 cup raw, unsalted almonds
- 2 ounces dark chocolate (70% cacao or higher), chopped
- 1 teaspoon coconut oil (optional)

PreparationTime: 10 minutes

Cook Time: 5 minutes

Total Time: 15 minutes

Serves: 4 (1/4 cup per serving)

Directions:

1. Line a baking sheet with parchment paper.

2. In a small saucepan, melt the dark chocolate and coconut oil (if using) over low heat, stirring constantly until smooth.

3. Remove the pan from the heat and stir in the almonds until they are fully coated with the melted chocolate.

4. Scoop the chocolate-coated almond clusters onto the prepared baking sheet, spacing them apart.

5. Refrigerate the clusters for at least 5 minutes, or until the chocolate has hardened.

Storage Instructions:
The dark chocolate and almond clusters can be stored in an airtight container in the refrigerator for up to 1 week.

Variations and Tips:
- Use a combination of nuts, such as walnuts, pecans, or hazelnuts, instead of just almonds.
- Add a sprinkle of sea salt or a pinch of cinnamon to the melted chocolate for extra flavor.
- Drizzle a small amount of melted white chocolate over the top of the clusters for a decorative touch.

Nutrition Facts:
Calories: 150 - Total Fat: 12g - Saturated Fat: 4g - Cholesterol: 0mg
Sodium: 0mg - Total Carbohydrates: 8g - Dietary Fiber: 3g - Sugars: 4g - Protein: 4g

This snack is an excellent choice for managing type 2 diabetes. Dark chocolate is a rich source of antioxidants and can help to satisfy sweet cravings, while the almonds provide healthy fats and protein to help keep blood sugar levels stable. The combination of the fiber-rich nuts and the moderate amount of dark chocolate makes this a well-balanced snack that can support blood sugar management.

Desserts that Won't Spike Your Blood Sugar

85. Frozen Banana Bites with Peanut Butter

Ingredients:
- 1 medium banana, peeled and sliced into 8 rounds
- 2 tablespoons natural peanut butter

PreparationTime: 10 minutes
Cook Time: 0 minutes (freezing time: 2 hours)
Total Time: 2 hours 10 minutes

Serves: 4 (2 bites per serving)

Directions:

1. Spread a thin layer of peanut butter on one side of each banana slice.

2. Place the peanut butter-topped banana slices on a parchment-lined baking sheet.

3. Freeze the banana bites for at least 2 hours, or until completely frozen.

Storage Instructions:

The frozen banana bites can be stored in an airtight container in the freezer for up to 2 months.

Variations and Tips:
- Use different nut butters, such as almond or cashew butter, instead of peanut butter.
- Dip the frozen banana bites in melted dark chocolate for an extra treat.
- Sprinkle a small amount of cinnamon or a pinch of sea salt over the peanut butter before freezing.

Nutrition Facts:
Calories: 100
Total Fat: 6g
Saturated Fat: 1g
Cholesterol: 0mg
Sodium: 0mg
Total Carbohydrates: 10g
Dietary Fiber: 2g
Sugars: 6g
Protein: 3g

This snack is an excellent choice for managing type 2 diabetes. Bananas are a low-glycemic fruit that provide natural sweetness and fiber, which can help to slow the absorption of carbohydrates and keep blood sugar levels stable. The peanut butter adds healthy fats and protein, which can also help to regulate blood sugar. The combination of the fiber-rich banana and the protein-rich peanut butter makes this a well-balanced snack that can support blood sugar management.

Desserts that Won't Spike Your Blood Sugar

86. Almond Flour Brownies

Ingredients:
- 1 cup almond flour
- 1/4 cup unsweetened cocoa powder
- 1/4 teaspoon baking soda
- 1/4 teaspoon salt
- 1/2 cup granulated erythritol or other low-calorie sweetener
- 2 large eggs
- 1/4 cup melted coconut oil or unsalted butter
- 1 teaspoon vanilla extract

PreparationTime: 15 minutes
Cook Time: 25 minutes
Total Time: 40 minutes

Serves: 9 (1 brownie per serving)

Directions:
1. Preheat the oven to 350°F (175°C). Grease an 8x8-inch baking pan.
2. In a medium bowl, whisk together the almond flour, cocoa powder, baking soda, and salt.
3. In a separate bowl, beat the eggs and erythritol until well combined. Stir in the melted coconut oil or butter and vanilla extract.
4. Add the dry ingredients to the wet ingredients and mix until just combined, being careful not to overmix.
5. Spread the batter evenly into the prepared baking pan.
6. Bake for 22-25 minutes, or until a toothpick inserted in the center comes out clean.
7. Allow the brownies to cool completely before cutting into 9 squares.

Storage Instructions:
The almond flour brownies can be stored in an airtight container at room temperature for up to 5 days.

Variations and Tips:
- Add a sprinkle of chopped walnuts or pecans on top of the batter before baking for extra crunch.
- Drizzle a small amount of melted dark chocolate over the cooled brownies for a decadent touch.
- Substitute the erythritol with a different low-calorie sweetener, such as monk fruit or stevia, to suit your preferences.

Nutrition Facts:
Calories: 150 - Total Fat: 12g - Saturated Fat: 6g - Cholesterol: 35mg
Sodium: 105mg - Total Carbohydrates: 8g - Dietary Fiber: 3g - Sugars: 2g - Protein: 4g

These almond flour brownies are an excellent treat for managing type 2 diabetes. The use of almond flour and a low-calorie sweetener helps to keep the carbohydrate and sugar content low, while still providing a rich, chocolatey flavor. The healthy fats from the almond flour and coconut oil can also help to regulate blood sugar levels. Portion control is key, as these brownies should be enjoyed as an occasional treat within a balanced diet.

Desserts that Won't Spike Your Blood Sugar

87. Fresh Strawberries with Balsamic Reduction

Ingredients:
- 1 cup fresh strawberries, hulled and sliced
- 2 tablespoons balsamic vinegar
- 1 teaspoon honey (optional)

PreparationTime: 10 minutes

Cook Time: 10 minutes

Total Time: 20 minutes

Serves: 2 (1/2 cup strawberries per serving)

Directions:

1. In a small saucepan, bring the balsamic vinegar
to a simmer over medium heat. Reduce the heat to low and let the vinegar simmer for 8-10 minutes, or until it has reduced by about half and thickened slightly.
2. Remove the balsamic reduction from the heat and stir in the honey, if using. Allow it to cool slightly.
3. Arrange the sliced strawberries on a plate or in a small bowl.
4. Drizzle the warm balsamic reduction over the strawberries.

Storage Instructions:
The balsamic reduction can be stored in an airtight container in the refrigerator for up to 1 week. The strawberries can be stored in the refrigerator for up to 3-4 days.

Variations and Tips:
- Use different types of berries, such as raspberries or blackberries, instead of strawberries.
- Add a sprinkle of chopped fresh mint or a pinch of black pepper for extra flavor.
- Serve the strawberries and balsamic reduction with a small amount of plain Greek yogurt or a crumble of feta cheese.

Nutrition Facts:
Calories: 80
Total Fat: 0g
Saturated Fat: 0g
Cholesterol: 0mg
Sodium: 0mg
Total Carbohydrates: 18g
Dietary Fiber: 3g
Sugars: 14g
Protein: 1g

This snack is an excellent choice for managing type 2 diabetes. Strawberries are a low-glycemic fruit that provide fiber, vitamins, and antioxidants. The balsamic reduction adds a touch of sweetness and acidity, which can help to balance the natural sweetness of the strawberries. The combination of the fiber-rich fruit and the moderate amount of natural sweetener makes this a well-balanced snack that can support blood sugar management.

Desserts that Won't Spike Your Blood Sugar

88. Coconut Flour Cookies

Ingredients:
- 1 cup coconut flour
- 1/2 cup unsweetened shredded coconut
- 1/4 cup granulated sugar
- 1/4 cup unsalted butter, softened
- 1 large egg
- 1 teaspoon vanilla extract
- 1/4 teaspoon baking soda
- 1/4 teaspoon salt

PreparationTime: 10 minutes
Cook Time: 12 minutes
Total Time: 22 minutes
Serves: 12 cookies

Directions:
1. Preheat the oven to 350°F (175°C). Line a baking sheet with parchment paper.
2. In a medium bowl, whisk together the coconut flour, shredded coconut, sugar, baking soda, and salt.
3. In a separate bowl, beat the butter and vanilla extract until smooth. Beat in the egg until well combined.
4. Add the dry ingredients to the wet ingredients and mix until a dough forms.
5. Scoop the dough by the tablespoonful and place them on the prepared baking sheet, spacing them about 2 inches apart.
6. Bake for 10-12 minutes, or until the cookies are lightly golden around the edges.
7. Remove the cookies from the oven and let them cool on the baking sheet for 5 minutes before transferring them to a wire rack to cool completely.

Storage Instructions:
Store the cookies in an airtight container at room temperature for up to 1 week.

Variations and Tips:
- For a chewier cookie, add 1/4 cup of almond flour or coconut flour to the dough.
- Dip the cooled cookies in melted dark chocolate for a delicious treat.
- Sprinkle the cookies with a pinch of sea salt before baking for a sweet and salty flavor.
- Use coconut sugar instead of granulated sugar for a deeper caramel flavor.

Nutrition Facts:

Calories: 100
Total Fat: 7g
Saturated Fat: 5g
Cholesterol: 20mg
Sodium: 75mg
Total Carbohydrates: 8g
Dietary Fiber: 3g
Total Sugars: 4g
Protein: 2g

Desserts that Won't Spike Your Blood Sugar

89. Avocado Chocolate Mousse

Ingredients:
- 2 ripe avocados, pitted and flesh scooped out
- 1/2 cup unsweetened cocoa powder
- 1/4 cup maple syrup
- 1/4 cup unsweetened almond milk
- 1 teaspoon vanilla extract
- 1/4 teaspoon sea salt

PreparationTime: 15 minutes
Chilling Time: 2 hours
Total Time: 2 hours 15 minutes
Serves: 4

Directions:

1. In a food processor or high-speed blender, combine the avocado flesh, cocoa powder, maple syrup, almond milk, vanilla extract, and sea salt. Blend until smooth and creamy, scraping down the sides as needed.

2. Transfer the mousse to a bowl or individual serving dishes. Cover and refrigerate for at least 2 hours, or until chilled and set.

3. Serve the avocado chocolate mousse chilled, garnished with fresh berries, shaved dark chocolate, or a sprinkle of cocoa powder, if desired.

Storage Instructions:
Store the avocado chocolate mousse in an airtight container in the refrigerator for up to 3 days.

Variations and Tips:
- For a richer flavor, use dark cocoa powder instead of unsweetened cocoa powder.
- Swap the maple syrup for honey or agave nectar.
- Add a pinch of cinnamon or a splash of espresso for a mocha-flavored mousse.
- Top the mousse with toasted coconut flakes, crushed nuts, or a drizzle of melted dark chocolate.

Nutrition Facts:

Calories: 180
Total Fat: 12g
Saturated Fat: 2g
Cholesterol: 0mg
Sodium: 120mg
Total Carbohydrates: 18g
Dietary Fiber: 7g
Total Sugars: 9g
Protein: 3g

Desserts that Won't Spike Your Blood Sugar

90. Mixed Berry Sorbet

Ingredients:
- 2 cups mixed berries
(such as raspberries, blackberries, and blueberries)
- 1/4 cup granulated erythritol or other low-calorie sweetener
- 2 tablespoons freshly squeezed lemon juice
- 1/4 cup water

PreparationTime: 15 minutes
Freezing Time: 4-6 hours
Total Time: 4 hours 15 minutes
Serves: 4

Directions:

1. In a medium saucepan, combine the mixed berries, erythritol, lemon juice, and water. Bring the mixture to a simmer over medium heat, stirring occasionally, until the sweetener has dissolved and the berries have released their juices, about 5 minutes.

2. Remove the saucepan from the heat and let the berry mixture cool to room temperature.

3. Transfer the cooled berry mixture to a blender or food processor and blend until smooth.

4. Pour the blended berry mixture into a shallow baking dish or a metal loaf pan. Cover and freeze for 4-6 hours, stirring the mixture every 30 minutes, until it reaches a sorbet-like consistency.

5. Scoop the mixed berry sorbet into serving dishes and enjoy immediately.

Storage Instructions:
Store the mixed berry sorbet in an airtight container in the freezer for up to 2 weeks.

Variations and Tips:
- Use a combination of your favorite berries, such as strawberries, raspberries, and blackberries.
- Add a splash of vodka or white wine for an adult-friendly version.
- Garnish the sorbet with fresh mint leaves or a sprinkle of chopped nuts.
- For a creamier texture, add a tablespoon of full-fat coconut milk or Greek yogurt to the berry mixture before blending.

Nutrition Facts:

Calories: 80 - Total Fat: 0g - Saturated Fat: 0g - Cholesterol: 0mg - Sodium: 5mg
Total Carbohydrates: 18g - Dietary Fiber: 4g - Total Sugars: 10g - Protein: 1g

This mixed berry sorbet is a refreshing and low-calorie dessert option that is suitable for managing type 2 diabetes. The use of erythritol, a low-calorie sweetener, helps to keep the sugar content low, while the berries provide a good source of antioxidants and fiber.

Desserts that Won't Spike Your Blood Sugar

91. Baked Pear with Almonds

Ingredients:
- 4 ripe but firm pears, halved and cored
- 2 tablespoons unsalted butter, melted
- 2 tablespoons chopped raw almonds
- 2 tablespoons granulated erythritol or other low-calorie sweetener
- 1 teaspoon ground cinnamon
- 1/4 teaspoon ground nutmeg

PreparationTime: 10 minutes
Baking Time: 25 minutes
Total Time: 35 minutes
Serves: 4

Directions:
1. Preheat the oven to 375°F (190°C). Line a baking sheet with parchment paper.

2. Place the pear halves, cut-side up, on the prepared baking sheet.

3. In a small bowl, combine the melted butter, chopped almonds, erythritol, cinnamon, and nutmeg. Mix well.

4. Spoon the almond mixture evenly over the pear halves, making sure to fill the cored centers.

5. Bake for 20-25 minutes, or until the pears are tender and the almond topping is lightly golden.

6. Remove the baked pears from the oven and let them cool for a few minutes before serving.

Storage Instructions:
Store any leftover baked pears in an airtight container in the refrigerator for up to 3 days.

Variations and Tips:
- For a crunchy topping, add a tablespoon of chopped walnuts or pecans to the almond mixture.
- Drizzle a small amount of unsweetened almond milk or Greek yogurt over the baked pears before serving.
- Sprinkle a pinch of ground ginger or cardamom along with the cinnamon and nutmeg for added warmth.
- Serve the baked pears warm or at room temperature, with a scoop of low-sugar vanilla ice cream or a dollop of whipped cream, if desired.

Nutrition Facts:

Calories: 150 - Total Fat: 8g - Saturated Fat: 3g - Cholesterol: 10mg
Sodium: 5mg - Total Carbohydrates: 20g - Dietary Fiber: 4g - Total Sugars: 10g - Protein: 2g

This baked pear with almonds recipe is a delicious and healthy dessert option for those managing type 2 diabetes. The use of erythritol as a sweetener helps to keep the sugar content low, while the pears and almonds provide fiber, healthy fats, and essential nutrients.

Desserts that Won't Spike Your Blood Sugar

92. Sugar-Free Lemon Cheesecake

Ingredients:
Crust:
- 1 1/2 cups almond flour
- 2 tablespoons unsalted butter, melted
- 1 tablespoon granulated erythritol or other low-calorie sweetener

Filling:
- 24 ounces (680g) full-fat cream cheese, softened
- 3/4 cup granulated erythritol or other low-calorie sweetener
- 2 large eggs
- 1/4 cup freshly squeezed lemon juice
- 1 tablespoon grated lemon zest
- 1 teaspoon vanilla extract
- 1/4 teaspoon salt

PreparationTime: 20 minutes
Baking Time: 55 minutes
Chilling Time: 4 hours
Total Time: 5 hours 15 minutes
Serves: 8

Directions:
1. Preheat the oven to 325°F (165°C). Grease a 9-inch springform pan.
2. In a medium bowl, mix together the almond flour, melted butter, and erythritol for the crust. Press the mixture evenly into the bottom of the prepared springform pan.
3. In a large bowl, beat the cream cheese with an electric mixer until smooth and creamy. Gradually add the erythritol and beat until well combined.
4. Add the eggs one at a time, beating well after each addition. Stir in the lemon juice, lemon zest, vanilla extract, and salt until the filling is smooth and well blended.
5. Pour the cheesecake filling over the prepared crust and smooth the top.
6. Bake for 50-55 minutes, or until the center is almost set. The cheesecake should still have a slight jiggle in the center.
7. Turn off the oven and leave the cheesecake inside with the door slightly ajar for 1 hour.
8. Remove the cheesecake from the oven and let it cool completely on a wire rack, then refrigerate for at least 4 hours or overnight before serving.

Storage Instructions:
Store the sugar-free lemon cheesecake in the refrigerator for up to 5 days.

Variations and Tips:
- For a creamier texture, use full-fat Greek yogurt in place of some of the cream cheese.
- Top the chilled cheesecake with fresh berries or a sugar-free fruit compote.
- Sprinkle the top of the cheesecake with a dusting of powdered erythritol or a few lemon zest curls.
- Experiment with different low-calorie sweeteners, such as monk fruit or stevia, to find your preferred taste.

Desserts that Won't Spike Your Blood Sugar

93. Pumpkin Pie with Almond Crust

Ingredients:
Crust:
- 1 1/2 cups almond flour
- 2 tablespoons unsalted butter, melted
- 1 tablespoon granulated erythritol or
other low-calorie sweetener

Filling:
- 1 (15-ounce) can pumpkin puree
- 3 large eggs
- 3/4 cup unsweetened almond milk
- 1/2 cup granulated erythritol or other low-calorie sweetener
- 1 teaspoon ground cinnamon
- 1/2 teaspoon ground ginger
- 1/4 teaspoon ground nutmeg
- 1/4 teaspoon ground cloves
- 1/4 teaspoon salt

PreparationTime: 20 minutes
Baking Time: 50 minutes
Cooling Time: 2 hours
Total Time: 2 hours 70 minutes
Serves: 8

Directions:
1. Preheat the oven to 350°F (175°C). Grease a 9-inch pie dish.

2. In a medium bowl, mix together the almond flour, melted butter, and erythritol for the crust. Press the mixture evenly into the bottom and up the sides of the prepared pie dish.

3. In a large bowl, whisk together the pumpkin puree, eggs, almond milk, erythritol, cinnamon, ginger, nutmeg, cloves, and salt until well combined.

4. Pour the pumpkin filling into the prepared almond crust.

5. Bake for 45-50 minutes, or until the center is almost set. The pie should still have a slight jiggle in the center.

6. Remove the pie from the oven and let it cool completely on a wire rack, about 2 hours.

7. Refrigerate the pumpkin pie for at least 2 hours before serving.

Storage Instructions:
Store the pumpkin pie in the refrigerator for up to 4 days.

Variations and Tips:
- For a creamier texture, use full-fat coconut milk or heavy cream instead of almond milk.
- Top the chilled pie with a dollop of unsweetened whipped cream or a sprinkle of chopped toasted pecans.
- Experiment with different low-calorie sweeteners, such as monk fruit or stevia, to find your preferred taste.
- Add a teaspoon of vanilla extract to the filling for extra flavor.

Desserts that Won't Spike Your Blood Sugar

94. Chocolate Avocado Pudding

Ingredients:
- 2 ripe avocados, pitted and flesh scooped out
- 1/2 cup unsweetened cocoa powder
- 1/4 cup granulated erythritol or other low-calorie sweetener
- 1/4 cup unsweetened almond milk
- 1 teaspoon vanilla extract
- 1/4 teaspoon sea salt

Preparation Time: 10 minutes
Chilling Time: 2 hours
Total Time: 2 hours 10 minutes
Serves: 4

Directions:
1. In a food processor or high-speed blender, combine the avocado flesh, cocoa powder, erythritol, almond milk, vanilla extract, and sea salt. Blend until smooth and creamy, scraping down the sides as needed.
2. Transfer the chocolate avocado pudding to a bowl or individual serving dishes. Cover and refrigerate for at least 2 hours, or until chilled and set.
3. Serve the chocolate avocado pudding chilled, garnished with a sprinkle of cocoa powder, chopped nuts, or fresh berries, if desired.

Storage Instructions:
Store the chocolate avocado pudding in an airtight container in the refrigerator for up to 3 days.

Variations and Tips:
- For a richer flavor, use dark cocoa powder instead of unsweetened cocoa powder.
- Swap the almond milk for unsweetened coconut milk or cashew milk.
- Add a pinch of cinnamon or a splash of espresso for a mocha-flavored pudding.
- Top the pudding with toasted coconut flakes, crushed nuts, or a drizzle of sugar-free chocolate syrup.
- Freeze the pudding in popsicle molds for a refreshing, low-carb treat.

Nutrition Facts:

Calories: 180
Total Fat: 14g
Saturated Fat: 2g
Cholesterol: 0mg
Sodium: 120mg
Total Carbohydrates: 14g
Dietary Fiber: 8g
Total Sugars: 2g
Protein: 4g

This chocolate avocado pudding is a delicious and nutritious dessert option for those managing type 2 diabetes. The use of avocado and erythritol as a sweetener helps to keep the carbohydrate and sugar content low, while providing a rich and creamy texture.

Desserts that Won't Spike Your Blood Sugar

95. Ricotta Cheese with Fresh Figs

Ingredients:
- 1 cup full-fat ricotta cheese
- 2 tablespoons granulated erythritol or other low-calorie sweetener
- 1/2 teaspoon vanilla extract
- 4 fresh figs, quartered

PreparationTime: 5 minutes
Total Time: 5 minutes
Serves: 2

Directions:
1. In a small bowl, mix together the ricotta cheese, erythritol, and vanilla extract until well combined.

2. Divide the ricotta mixture between two serving bowls or plates.

3. Top each serving with the quartered fresh figs.

Storage Instructions:
Store any leftover ricotta and fig mixture in an airtight container in the refrigerator for up to 3 days.

Variations and Tips:
- For a creamier texture, use part-skim or whole-milk ricotta cheese.
- Drizzle a small amount of unsweetened almond milk or a touch of honey over the ricotta and figs.
- Sprinkle a pinch of cinnamon or a few chopped toasted almonds on top for added flavor and crunch.
- Use a variety of fresh figs, such as black mission, brown turkey, or green Kadota, for a colorful presentation.
- Serve the ricotta and fig mixture as a light dessert or a healthy snack.

Nutrition Facts:

Calories: 200
Total Fat: 12g
Saturated Fat: 7g
Cholesterol: 40mg
Sodium: 120mg
Total Carbohydrates: 14g
Dietary Fiber: 3g
Total Sugars: 10g
Protein: 12g

This ricotta cheese with fresh figs is a simple and delicious option for those managing type 2 diabetes. The use of erythritol as a sweetener helps to keep the sugar content low, while the ricotta cheese and figs provide a good source of protein, fiber, and essential nutrients.

Desserts that Won't Spike Your Blood Sugar

96. Cinnamon-Spiced Quinoa Pudding

Ingredients:
- 1 cup uncooked quinoa, rinsed
- 2 cups unsweetened almond milk
- 1/4 cup granulated erythritol or other low-calorie sweetener
- 1 teaspoon ground cinnamon
- 1/4 teaspoon ground nutmeg
- 1/4 teaspoon salt
- 1 teaspoon vanilla extract
- 1/4 cup chopped toasted almonds (optional)

PreparationTime: 10 minutes
Cooking Time: 25 minutes
Chilling Time: 2 hours
Total Time: 2 hours 35 minutes
Serves: 4

Directions:
1. In a medium saucepan, combine the rinsed quinoa and almond milk. Bring the mixture to a boil over medium-high heat.
2. Reduce the heat to low, cover the saucepan, and simmer for 15-20 minutes, or until the quinoa is tender and the liquid is mostly absorbed.
3. Remove the saucepan from the heat and stir in the erythritol, cinnamon, nutmeg, salt, and vanilla extract. Mix well until the sweetener is dissolved.
4. Transfer the cinnamon-spiced quinoa pudding to a bowl or individual serving dishes. Cover and refrigerate for at least 2 hours, or until chilled and thickened.
5. Serve the quinoa pudding chilled, garnished with the chopped toasted almonds, if desired.

Storage Instructions: Store the cinnamon-spiced quinoa pudding in an airtight container in the refrigerator for up to 4 days.

Variations and Tips:
- For a creamier texture, use full-fat coconut milk or a combination of almond milk and heavy cream.
- Add a tablespoon of chia seeds or ground flaxseed to the pudding for extra fiber and nutrients.
- Stir in a handful of fresh berries, such as raspberries or blueberries, for a pop of color and flavor.
- Top the chilled pudding with a sprinkle of unsweetened shredded coconut or a drizzle of sugar-free caramel sauce.
- Experiment with different low-calorie sweeteners, such as monk fruit or stevia, to find your preferred taste.

Nutrition Facts:

Calories: 180 - Total Fat: 6g - Saturated Fat: 1g - Cholesterol: 0mg - Sodium: 160mg
Total Carbohydrates: 25g - Dietary Fiber: 4g - Total Sugars: 4g - Protein: 6g

This cinnamon-spiced quinoa pudding is a delightful and nutritious dessert option for those managing type 2 diabetes. The use of quinoa and erythritol as a sweetener helps to keep the carbohydrate and sugar content low, while providing a satisfying and comforting treat.

Desserts that Won't Spike Your Blood Sugar

97. Low-Carb Raspberry Cheesecake Bars

Ingredients:
Crust:
- 1 1/2 cups almond flour
- 2 tablespoons unsalted butter, melted
- 1 tablespoon granulated erythritol or other low-calorie sweetener

Filling:
- 16 ounces (450g) full-fat cream cheese, softened
- 1/2 cup granulated erythritol or other low-calorie sweetener
- 2 large eggs
- 1 teaspoon vanilla extract
- 1/4 teaspoon salt
- 1 cup fresh or frozen raspberries

PreparationTime: 20 minutes
Baking Time: 30 minutes
Chilling Time: 2 hours
Total Time: 2 hours 50 minutes
Serves: 12 bars

Directions:
1. Preheat the oven to 325°F (165°C). Grease an 8x8-inch baking pan and line it with parchment paper, leaving some overhang on the sides for easy removal.
2. In a medium bowl, mix together the almond flour, melted butter, and erythritol for the crust. Press the mixture evenly into the bottom of the prepared baking pan.
3. In a large bowl, beat the cream cheese with an electric mixer until smooth and creamy. Gradually add the erythritol and beat until well combined.
4. Add the eggs one at a time, beating well after each addition. Stir in the vanilla extract and salt until the filling is smooth and well blended.
5. Gently fold in the fresh or frozen raspberries.
6. Pour the cheesecake filling over the prepared crust and smooth the top.
7. Bake for 25-30 minutes, or until the center is almost set. The bars should still have a slight jiggle in the center.
8. Remove the bars from the oven and let them cool completely on a wire rack, then refrigerate for at least 2 hours before cutting and serving.

Storage Instructions:
Store the low-carb raspberry cheesecake bars in the refrigerator for up to 5 days.

Variations and Tips:
- For a creamier texture, use full-fat Greek yogurt in place of some of the cream cheese.
- Swap the raspberries for other low-carb berries, such as blackberries or blueberries.
- Drizzle the chilled bars with a sugar-free raspberry or chocolate sauce.
- Sprinkle the top of the bars with a dusting of powdered erythritol or a few fresh raspberry halves.
- Experiment with different low-calorie sweeteners, such as monk fruit or stevia, to find your preferred taste.

Desserts that Won't Spike Your Blood Sugar

98. Zucchini Bread with Walnuts

Ingredients:
- 1 1/2 cups almond flour
- 1/2 cup coconut flour
- 1 teaspoon baking powder
- 1/2 teaspoon baking soda
- 1/2 teaspoon ground cinnamon
- 1/4 teaspoon ground nutmeg
- 1/4 teaspoon salt
- 3 large eggs
- 1/2 cup granulated erythritol or other low-calorie sweetener
- 1/4 cup unsweetened applesauce
- 1/4 cup avocado oil or melted coconut oil
- 1 teaspoon vanilla extract
- 1 1/2 cups grated zucchini (about 1 medium zucchini)
- 1/2 cup chopped walnuts

PreparationTime: 15 minutes
Baking Time: 55 minutes
Total Time: 1 hour 10 minutes
Serves: 12 slices

Directions:
1. Preheat the oven to 350°F (175°C). Grease a 9x5-inch loaf pan and line it with parchment paper, leaving some overhang on the sides for easy removal.
2. In a medium bowl, whisk together the almond flour, coconut flour, baking powder, baking soda, cinnamon, nutmeg, and salt.
3. In a separate large bowl, beat the eggs and erythritol until well combined. Stir in the applesauce, oil, and vanilla extract.
4. Add the dry ingredients to the wet ingredients and mix until just combined. Fold in the grated zucchini and chopped walnuts.
5. Pour the batter into the prepared loaf pan and smooth the top.
6. Bake for 50-55 minutes, or until a toothpick inserted into the center comes out clean.
7. Allow the zucchini bread to cool in the pan for 10 minutes, then use the parchment paper to lift it out and transfer it to a wire rack to cool completely.

Storage Instructions:
Store the zucchini bread in an airtight container at room temperature for up to 4 days, or in the refrigerator for up to 1 week.

Variations and Tips:
- For a moister texture, replace the applesauce with unsweetened pumpkin puree or mashed ripe banana.
- Add a handful of chopped pecans or sliced almonds in addition to the walnuts.
- Stir in a tablespoon of ground flaxseed or chia seeds for extra fiber and nutrients.
- Drizzle the cooled bread with a sugar-free cream cheese glaze or a dusting of powdered erythritol.
- Experiment with different low-calorie sweeteners, such as monk fruit or stevia, to find your preferred taste.

Desserts that Won't Spike Your Blood Sugar

99. Sugar-Free Chocolate Chip Cookies

Ingredients:
- 1 1/2 cups almond flour
- 1/2 cup coconut flour
- 1/2 teaspoon baking soda
- 1/4 teaspoon salt
- 1/2 cup unsalted butter, softened
- 1/2 cup granulated erythritol or other low-calorie sweetener
- 1 large egg
- 1 teaspoon vanilla extract
- 1/2 cup sugar-free dark chocolate chips or chopped sugar-free dark chocolate

PreparationTime: 15 minutes
Baking Time: 12 minutes
Total Time: 27 minutes
Serves: 18 cookies

Directions:
1. Preheat the oven to 350°F (175°C). Line a baking sheet with parchment paper.
2. In a medium bowl, whisk together the almond flour, coconut flour, baking soda, and salt.
3. In a large bowl, beat the softened butter and erythritol until light and fluffy. Beat in the egg and vanilla extract until well combined.
4. Gradually add the dry ingredients to the wet ingredients and mix until a dough forms. Fold in the sugar-free chocolate chips.
5. Scoop the dough by the tablespoonful and place them on the prepared baking sheet, spacing them about 2 inches apart.
6. Bake for 10-12 minutes, or until the cookies are lightly golden around the edges.
7. Remove the cookies from the oven and let them cool on the baking sheet for 5 minutes before transferring them to a wire rack to cool completely.

Storage Instructions:
Store the sugar-free chocolate chip cookies in an airtight container at room temperature for up to 1 week.

Variations and Tips:
- For a chewier cookie, add 1/4 cup of almond butter or peanut butter to the dough.
- Sprinkle a pinch of sea salt on top of the cookies before baking for a sweet and salty flavor.
- Use a combination of sugar-free chocolate chips and chopped nuts, such as pecans or walnuts, for added texture and crunch.
- Experiment with different low-calorie sweeteners, such as monk fruit or stevia, to find your preferred taste.
- Chill the dough for 30 minutes before baking for a thicker, chewier cookie.

Nutrition Facts:

Calories: 110 - Total Fat: 9g - Saturated Fat: 3g - Cholesterol: 15mg - Sodium: 75mg
Total Carbohydrates: 6g - Dietary Fiber: 3g - Total Sugars: 1g - Protein: 3g

Desserts that Won't Spike Your Blood Sugar

100. Almond Butter and Coconut Balls

Ingredients:
- 1 cup unsweetened almond butter
- 1/4 cup granulated erythritol or other low-calorie sweetener
- 1/4 cup unsweetened shredded coconut, plus more for rolling
- 1 teaspoon vanilla extract
- 1/4 teaspoon sea salt

PreparationTime: 10 minutes
Chilling Time: 30 minutes
Total Time: 40 minutes
Serves: 12 balls

Directions:

1. In a medium bowl, stir together the almond butter, erythritol, 1/4 cup of shredded coconut, vanilla extract, and sea salt until well combined.

2. Using a tablespoon or small cookie scoop, form the mixture into 12 equal-sized balls.

3. Roll the balls in the additional shredded coconut to coat them completely.

4. Place the coated balls on a parchment-lined baking sheet and refrigerate for at least 30 minutes to allow them to firm up.

Storage Instructions:
Store the almond butter and coconut balls in an airtight container in the refrigerator for up to 1 week.

Variations and Tips:
- For a crunchy texture, add 2 tablespoons of chopped toasted almonds or pecans to the almond butter mixture.
- Drizzle the chilled balls with a small amount of melted sugar-free dark chocolate for a decadent treat.
- Roll the balls in a mixture of shredded coconut and ground cinnamon or cocoa powder for a different flavor profile.
- Substitute peanut butter or cashew butter for the almond butter, if desired.
- Freeze the balls for up to 3 months and thaw in the refrigerator before serving.

Nutrition Facts:

Calories: 130 - Total Fat: 11g - Saturated Fat: 3g - Cholesterol: 0mg
Sodium: 75mg - Total Carbohydrates: 5g - Dietary Fiber: 3g - Total Sugars: 1g - Protein: 4g

These almond butter and coconut balls are a delicious and nutritious snack or dessert option for those managing type 2 diabetes. The use of almond butter and erythritol as a sweetener helps to keep the carbohydrate and sugar content low, while the coconut provides a satisfying texture and flavor.

Desserts that Won't Spike Your Blood Sugar

Chapter 9: Meal Planning Tips for One Person

Meal planning is a critical component of managing type 2 diabetes effectively. It helps ensure you maintain a balanced diet, keep blood sugar levels stable, and avoid the pitfalls of last-minute unhealthy food choices. For those living alone, meal planning can be particularly beneficial as it minimizes food waste, saves time, and reduces the stress of daily meal preparation. This chapter provides practical tips and strategies for successful meal planning tailored for one person.

Benefits of Meal Planning

Meal planning offers numerous advantages, including:

- Improved Blood Sugar Control: By planning meals ahead of time, you can ensure they are balanced and contain the appropriate mix of carbohydrates, proteins, and fats to keep your blood sugar levels stable.

- Reduced Food Waste: Planning meals helps you buy only what you need, which is especially important when cooking for one.

- Time and Money Savings: Preparing a shopping list based on your meal plan can save you time in the grocery store and reduce impulse purchases.

- Stress Reduction: Knowing what you will eat each day eliminates the daily decision-making process and reduces stress.

Steps for Effective Meal Planning

- Assess Your Nutritional Needs: Understand the dietary guidelines for managing type 2 diabetes. Focus on incorporating whole grains, lean proteins, healthy fats, and plenty of fruits and vegetables into your meals.

- Plan Your Meals for the Week: Start by planning breakfast, lunch, dinner, and snacks for the entire week. Consider your schedule and plan for days when you might need quicker, easier meals.

- Create a Shopping List: Once your meals are planned, make a detailed shopping list. This will help you stay organized and ensure you have all the ingredients you need.

- Batch Cooking and Prepping: Prepare ingredients in advance to save time during the week. For example, chop vegetables, cook grains, and portion out snacks.

- Storage and Portion Control: Invest in good-quality storage containers to keep your meals fresh. Use these containers to portion out meals and snacks, making it easy to grab and go.

Sample Meal Plan for One Person

Here's a sample meal plan for a week, tailored for one person managing type 2 diabetes:

Monday
- Breakfast: Spinach and Feta Omelette
- Lunch: Grilled Chicken Salad with Mixed Greens and Avocado
- Dinner: Baked Salmon with Quinoa and Steamed Broccoli
- Snack: Apple Slices with Almond Butter

Tuesday
- Breakfast: Greek Yogurt with Berries and Chia Seeds
- Lunch: Lentil Soup with Carrots and Celery
- Dinner: Chicken Stir-Fry with Snap Peas and Brown Rice
- Snack: Carrot Sticks with Hummus

Wednesday
- Breakfast: Oatmeal with Almond Butter and Sliced Bananas
- Lunch: Turkey and Spinach Wrap
- Dinner: Baked Cod with Lemon and Dill
- Snack: Greek Yogurt with Cucumber Slices

Thursday
- Breakfast: Avocado Toast with Poached Egg
- Lunch: Quinoa Salad with Chickpeas and Feta
- Dinner: Turkey Meatballs with Zucchini Noodles
- Snack: Mixed Nuts and Seeds

Friday
- Breakfast: Smoothie Bowl with Spinach, Avocado, and Flax Seeds
- Lunch: Vegetable Stir-Fry with Tofu and Brown Rice
- Dinner: Beef and Vegetable Kebabs
- Snack: Edamame with Sea Salt

Saturday
- Breakfast: Cottage Cheese with Fresh Peaches and Cinnamon
- Lunch: Tuna Salad with Olive Oil and Lemon Dressing
- Dinner: Stuffed Bell Peppers with Ground Turkey and Quinoa
- Snack: Cottage Cheese with Pineapple Chunks

Sunday
- Breakfast: Whole Grain Pancakes with Blueberries
- Lunch: Roasted Beet and Goat Cheese Salad
- Dinner: Grilled Salmon with Asparagus
- Snack: Cherry Tomatoes with Mozzarella Balls

Grocery Shopping Tips

- Buy in Small Quantities: Purchase perishable items in smaller quantities to ensure they stay fresh and minimize waste.

- Choose Versatile Ingredients: Select ingredients that can be used in multiple recipes. For example, spinach can be used in omelets, salads, and smoothies.

- Frozen and Canned Options: Stock up on frozen vegetables and canned beans, which have a longer shelf life and can be convenient for quick meals.

Batch Cooking Tips

- Cook Staples in Bulk: Prepare staples like brown rice, quinoa, and grilled chicken in large batches and store them in the refrigerator or freezer for easy access.

- Portion and Freeze: Portion out meals and freeze them in individual servings. This makes it easy to reheat a healthy meal when you don't have time to cook.

- Label and Date: Always label and date your containers to keep track of what you have and when it was prepared.

Staying Motivated

- Set Realistic Goals: Start with small, achievable goals and gradually build up your meal planning skills.

- Keep It Interesting: Try new recipes and rotate your meals to keep things interesting and prevent boredom.

- Celebrate Successes: Reward yourself for sticking to your meal plan and making healthy choices. Positive reinforcement can keep you motivated.

Meal planning is a powerful tool for managing type 2 diabetes, especially for those cooking for one. By taking the time to plan your meals, create a shopping list, and prepare ingredients in advance, you can ensure that you always have healthy, diabetes-friendly meals on hand. This proactive approach will help you maintain stable blood sugar levels, reduce stress, and enjoy a varied and nutritious diet.

Strategies for Eating Out with Type 2 Diabetes

Eating out can be a delightful experience, offering a break from cooking and an opportunity to enjoy different cuisines. However, for individuals managing type 2 diabetes, it can present certain challenges. Restaurant meals often come in large portions and may contain hidden sugars, unhealthy fats, and excessive carbohydrates, all of which can affect blood sugar levels. This chapter provides practical strategies for enjoying restaurant meals while maintaining control over your diabetes.

Pre-Meal Preparation
Before heading to a restaurant, it's beneficial to do some preparation:

- Research the Menu: Many restaurants provide their menus online. Look for dishes that fit your dietary needs and note any questions you might have about preparation methods or ingredients.

- Check Nutritional Information: Some establishments offer nutritional information for their dishes. Use this data to choose meals that align with your diabetes management plan.

- Eat a Small Snack: Eating a small, healthy snack before dining out can help you avoid overeating at the restaurant.

Choosing a Restaurant
Select a restaurant that offers a variety of healthy options:

1. Ethnic Cuisines: Mediterranean, Japanese, and Thai restaurants often provide a range of healthy choices that include lean proteins, vegetables, and whole grains.
2. Farm-to-Table: These restaurants focus on fresh, locally sourced ingredients and often have healthier menu items.
3. Salad Bars: Restaurants with salad bars can be a good choice as they allow you to control the ingredients and portion sizes.

Ordering Tips
When ordering, consider the following tips to help manage your blood sugar levels:

1. Ask Questions: Don't hesitate to ask the server about how dishes are prepared. Request modifications such as grilling instead of frying or serving sauces on the side.
2. Control Portions: Restaurant portions are often larger than necessary. Consider sharing a meal with a friend or ask for a to-go box and portion out half of your meal before you start eating.
3. Choose Wisely: Opt for dishes that include plenty of vegetables, lean proteins, and whole grains. Avoid items that are fried, breaded, or smothered in creamy sauces.
4. Watch the Carbs: Be mindful of carbohydrate-heavy foods like bread, pasta, and rice. If you indulge, try to balance it with lower-carb choices.

Specific Cuisine Strategies

Different types of cuisine present unique challenges and opportunities for managing diabetes:

Italian Cuisine
- Opt for Whole Grain Pasta: If available, choose whole grain pasta or ask if the restaurant can substitute it.
- Choose Tomato-Based Sauces: These are generally lower in fat and calories compared to cream-based sauces.
- Mind the Bread: Italian restaurants often serve bread before the meal. Limit yourself to one small piece or skip it altogether.

Mexican Cuisine
- Go for Tacos: Soft corn tacos are a better choice than fried items like chimichangas or nachos.
- Load Up on Veggies: Add extra vegetables to your meal and choose guacamole or salsa instead of sour cream and cheese.
- Skip the Chips: Limit the consumption of tortilla chips, which are often high in carbs and calories.

Asian Cuisine
- Choose Stir-Fried or Steamed: Opt for dishes that are stir-fried or steamed rather than fried or battered.
- Ask for Brown Rice: If brown rice is available, choose it over white rice.
- Soy Sauce: Use low-sodium soy sauce to reduce sodium intake, which is often high in Asian cuisine.

Managing Desserts
Desserts can be particularly challenging, but you can still enjoy a sweet treat occasionally:
- Share a Dessert: Share a dessert with a friend to keep portion sizes small.
- Opt for Fruit: Fresh fruit or fruit-based desserts are often healthier options.
- Ask for Modifications: Request desserts with less sugar or ask if they can be prepared in a healthier way.

Alcohol Consumption
If you choose to drink alcohol, do so in moderation and with caution:
- Limit to One Drink: Stick to one alcoholic beverage per day for women and two for men.
- Choose Wisely: Opt for light beer, wine, or spirits mixed with soda water rather than sugary cocktails.
- Never Drink on an Empty Stomach: Consuming alcohol on an empty stomach can cause blood sugar levels to fluctuate unpredictably.

Eating out with type 2 diabetes doesn't mean you have to sacrifice enjoyment or flavor. With careful planning, informed choices, and mindful eating, you can dine out while keeping your blood sugar levels under control. By using the strategies outlined in this chapter, you can confidently navigate restaurant menus and enjoy meals out without compromising your health.

Benefits of Exercise for Type 2 Diabetes

Understanding the benefits of exercise can serve as a powerful motivator:

- Improved Blood Sugar Control: Exercise helps muscles use glucose more efficiently, reducing blood sugar levels.

- Increased Insulin Sensitivity: Regular activity enhances your body's response to insulin, making it easier to manage diabetes.

- Weight Management: Physical activity helps burn calories, aiding in weight loss and maintenance.

- Cardiovascular Health: Exercise strengthens the heart and improves circulation, reducing the risk of heart disease.

- Mental Health: Physical activity releases endorphins, which can help reduce stress, anxiety, and depression.

Types of Exercise

Different types of exercise offer various benefits. Incorporating a mix can keep your routine balanced and engaging:

- Aerobic Exercise: Activities like walking, jogging, cycling, and swimming increase heart rate and improve cardiovascular health. Aim for at least 150 minutes of moderate aerobic activity per week.

- Strength Training: Lifting weights or using resistance bands builds muscle mass, which helps the body burn more calories and improves insulin sensitivity. Include strength training exercises at least twice a week.

- Flexibility and Balance: Activities like yoga, Pilates, and stretching improve flexibility, balance, and reduce the risk of injury. Incorporate these exercises a few times a week.

- Interval Training: Alternating short bursts of intense activity with periods of rest or low-intensity exercise can improve cardiovascular fitness and glucose metabolism.

Incorporating exercise into your daily routine is essential for managing type 2 diabetes effectively. By understanding the benefits, choosing the right types of exercise, and overcoming common barriers, you can make physical activity a regular and enjoyable part of your life. Consistent exercise, combined with a balanced diet and regular blood sugar monitoring, will help you maintain control over your diabetes and improve your overall health and well-being.